MILK, MONEY, AND MADNESS

The Culture and Politics of Breastfeeding

Naomi Baumslag, M.D., M.P.H.
and
Dia L. Michels

Foreword by Dr. Richard Jolly,
Acting Executive Director, UNICEF

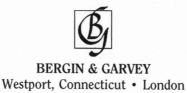

BERGIN & GARVEY
Westport, Connecticut • London

Library of Congress Cataloging-in-Publication Data

Baumslag, Naomi.
    Milk, money, and madness : the culture and politics of
breastfeeding / Naomi Baumslag and Dia L. Michels ; foreword by Dr. Richard Jolly.
        p. cm.
    Includes bibliographical references and index.
    ISBN 0-89789-407-3 (hc : alk. paper)
    1. Breast feeding—Health aspects.   2. Breast feeding—Social
aspects.   3. Breast milk.   4. Infant formulas.   I. Michels, Dia L.
II. Title.
RJ216.B28   1995
649'.33—dc20   95-14975

British Library Cataloguing in Publication Data is available.

Library of Congress Catalog Card Number: 95-14975

ISBN: 0-89789-407-3

First published in 1995

Bergin & Garvey, 88 Post Road West, Westport, CT 06881
An imprint of Greenwood Publishing Group Inc.

Printed in the United States of America

The paper used in this book complies with the
Permanent Paper Standard issued by the National
Information Standards Organization (Z39.48–1984).

10 9 8 7 6 5 4 3 2

For Victor, Beth, Aaron, Ruth, and our lost son Barry.

—NB

For Akaela and Zaydek, my bosom buddies.

—DLM

And dedicated to the memory of James Grant, Cecily D. Williams, and Derrick B. Jelliffe, all of whom fought tirelessly for well over half a century to make the world a better place for women and children.

—NB and DLM

Contents

Illustrations

TABLES

Foreword

For as long as there are children, breastfeeding will occupy a central, irreplaceable position in their survival, development, and well-being, in the rights of mothers, in the stability of families, and even in the economy of nations and in the defense of a clean and safe environment. So it naturally follows that, for as long as there is breastfeeding, UNICEF will remain committed to its promotion, protection, and support. Few health behaviors are as fundamental to the development and care of our children as breastfeeding, and few health messages have received the unconditional support that the adage "breastfeeding is best" enjoys worldwide.

Even unanimous consensus about the comparative advantage of breastfeeding has not proven enough, however, to expose and erase the myths and misinformation that endanger its practice. In a modern world that has increasingly distanced itself from nature, the unique contribution of breastfeeding is still too often underestimated, its protections underrated, and its practice mismanaged in too many health systems worldwide. The only foolproof means of protecting breastfeeding is to ensure that every family, community, health worker, and policymaker has full access to factual, scientific, and unabridged information—both about the benefits of breastfeeding and also about the risks involved in foregoing the practice. UNICEF applauds the welcome addition of new literature to the world's far-too-meager store of objective research, historical facts, and scientific data on breastfeeding.

I commend the authors of *Milk, Money, and Madness* for the considerable contribution they have made by voicing their opinions, contributing their knowledge, stimulating debate, and challenging conventional wisdom.

Dr. Richard Jolly
Acting Executive Director
UNICEF

Preface

We wrote this book because we are deeply committed to breastfeeding. Women have the right to breastfeed without interference, yet because of changing cultural attitudes and practices in this society, the information on breastfeeding is insufficient at best, inaccurate at worst.

The aim of this book is to bring alive the history, the culture, the biology, and the politics of breastfeeding so women can appreciate the contribution of breastfeeding to the survival of our species. Breastfeeding is a vital part of womanhood and mothering, and not a confining form of servitude.

This is a *Why To* book—not a *How To* book. A few generations ago, there would have been no need for a *Why To* treatise on breastfeeding. Nursing one's child was universal and socially acceptable. Women attended women at births and shared with them their mothering folklore. With the medicalization of birth, this is no longer the case. Most American women do not breastfeed, and those who do typically abandon it within a matter of weeks. The women who do continue to breastfeed often do so in a cultural vacuum. In addition to living apart from family and community and having mothers who relied on bottle-feeding, many first-time mothers have never even seen a mother nursing. Because of this, breastfeeding is often accompanied by awkwardness, embarrassment, and anxiety.

There are, however, women who always breastfeed their children, nursing their newborns moments after the birth, then continuing to nurse for years. And while the number is statistically small, these women will not hesitate to tell you that breastfeeding is, by far, one of the most powerful, self-affirming, satisfying experiences of their life. To know that you are providing your child with a miracle food and medicine, while at the same time achieving an unmatched bond and sense of closeness, is a unique experience.

Yet, so often the subject of breastfeeding is presented to pregnant women as little more than one feeding option, only marginally different from formula-feeding, and strictly a matter of personal choice. This is largely due to the indolence and ignorance of health workers. But breastfeeding is not similar to formula-feeding. True, they are the only two substances capable of sustaining a newborn until s/he is old enough to eat solid foods. But that is where the similarity ends. Medically, nutritionally, immunologically, and emotionally, breastmilk and infant formula—breastfeeding and bottle-feeding—are entirely different and unrelated.

Everyone who studies breastmilk must come away convinced that this is a most amazing fluid. It is a substance as life sustaining and as inimitable as blood. This book is about choices and rights, because the lack of accurate information about breastfeeding makes it hard for women to understand how their right to breastfeed is manipulated by those who profit when they choose not to.

An appreciation of breastfeeding leads to an appreciation of the breast itself, a gland composed largely of fatty tissue. Unfortunately, too often it is seen as an object of sexual desire rather than as a fountain of utilitarian magnificence. The lack of appreciation for the breast reflects a lack of appreciation of the female as a person. When the fluid responsible for sustaining human life is seen as essentially identical to a canned powder produced in a factory, it is easy to see how the appreciation of the breast (and with it, the female body) has been lost. This book is also about reclaiming that appreciation.

Acknowledgments

Many people helped make this book a reality. Particular thanks go to Barbara Heiser, Beth Styer, and Carol Huotari, La Leche League; René Smit, CNM; Minda Lazarov, U.S. Committee for UNICEF; Karlyn Sturmer, Action for Corporate Accountability; Andrew Radford, Baby Milk Action; Judy Canahuatis, Wellstart; and Vergie Hughes, Director, National Capitol Lactation Center and Human Milk Bank, Georgetown University Medical Center.

Literature and insights were gleaned from many individuals, especially Gabrielle Palmer, Dr. Michael Latham, Peggy Fairchild, Fred Clarkson, Dr. Penny Van Esterik, Gayle Gibbons; and Liz Nugent, APHA Clearinghouse on Maternal and Infant Nutrition; Dr. Fred Zerfas, and Elizabeth Baldwin. Jan Lazarus, History of Medicine Division, National Library of Medicine, provided invaluable assistance for illustrations.

Special thanks go to our publisher, Bergin & Garvey, for helping us bring this book to the public, and particularly to Lynn Taylor, Lynn Flint, Kathleen Silloway, and Ann Newman. Finally, our husbands, Ralph E. Yodaiken and Tony Gualtieri, have been wonderfully supportive and provided much encouragement over the years as we worked on this book.

Thanks, too, go to all the women and men who make the promotion of breastfeeding part of their daily lives.

Introduction

Lactation is the very core of our identity; the process evolved even before gestation and each mammal has evolved, over the millennia, a milk unique to its requirements, its behavior and its environment. It is such a spectacular survival strategy that we call ourselves, after the mammary gland, mammals . . . animals that suckle their young.
—Gabrielle Palmer, *The Politics of Breastfeeding*, 1993

It is an irony that this book needed to be written. It wasn't that long ago that breastfeeding was as much a part of the maternal experience as pregnancy (Figure 0.1). Until the 1930s, practically all American infants were breastfed by either their mother or a wet nurse. Our grandmothers never thought twice about nursing their children. Now, many American women do think twice about it . . . and decide not to bother. Each year, 1.8 million new mothers in the United States elect not to even try nursing. Pediatricians overwhelmingly agree that breastfeeding is best for babies, yet in the United States today only 53% of all new mothers even attempt it, and most abandon it quickly. Just 1 in 5 infants receives any breastmilk at all at 20 weeks of age.

When women decide to feed formula, they often see it as a choice between two infant foods. Breastfeeding, though, is much more than a means of providing calories to a newborn. It is the focal point of infant health (Figure 0.2). It is a natural extension to the processes of pregnancy and childbirth. It is a truly beautiful interactive process whereby both mother and child work together to produce a living biological substance that nourishes the infant, protects both mother and child from a plethora of diseases, and establishes a warm and loving relationship between them. Nursing is not just about the action of feeding a child with one's breasts, it is about nurturing for mother and child. Conceiving and carrying a fetus connects

Figure 0.1
Breastfeeding Mothers from around the World

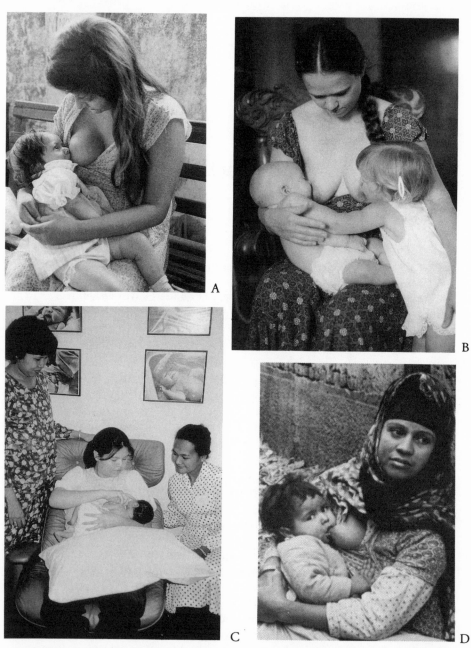

(A) Ecuador. *Photo courtesy*: UNICEF, neg. no. 8758. Photo by B. Wolff; (B) United States. Tandem Nursing. *Photo courtesy*: La Leche League International; (C) Thailand. *Photo courtesy*: Wellstart; (D) Egypt. *Photo courtesy*: UNICEF, neg. no. 8263. Photo by B. Wolff.

Figure 0.2
Breastfeeding—The Focal Point of Infant Health

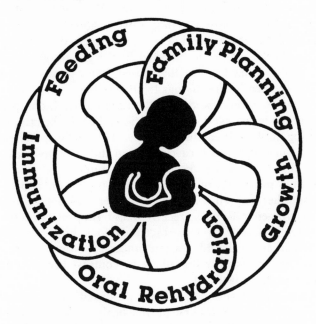

Breastfeeding is important for adequate growth: it provides against infections, prevents diarrhea, and is a natural form of family planning. *Source:* N. Baumslag, ed.
Breastfeeding: Passport to Life. NGO Committee on
UNICEF, Working Group on Nutrition, 1989.

a mother to her child genetically, but it is nurturing—and especially breastfeeding—that provides both mother and child with the powerful emotional
connection.

Breastfeeding is an unsentimental metaphor for how love works, in a way. You
don't decide how much or how deeply to love—you respond to the beloved, and
give with joy exactly as much as they want. (Marni Jackson, *The Mother Zone,*
1994)

Constant comparison of formula to breastmilk has succeeded in reducing
breastfeeding to the one-dimensional level of breastmilk substitutes. Infant
formula is just food, but the living fluid, called breastmilk, is food and
medicine uniquely engineered for human consumption. Breastfed babies are
healthier, have fewer hospitalizations, and have lower mortality rates than
formula-fed infants. They not only have fewer childhood ailments, they also

have less chronic illness throughout their lives. Far too many infants die each year in this country from diseases that breastmilk helps prevent—including diarrhea, sudden infant death syndrome (SIDS), and pneumonia.

Increasing Americans' breastfeeding rates would prevent a tremendous amount of childhood disease and death. The increased morbidity and mortality of formula-fed infants is reflected in the greater expenses for their health care. If every newborn in the United States were breastfed for just twelve weeks, the heath care savings from avoiding nonchronic diseases *in the first year of life* would be $2-4 billion annually. Not surprisingly, the Federal Government has established a national health objective for the year 2000 of raising national breastfeeding rates. The goal is to increase to 75% the number of new mothers breastfeeding in the early postpartum period, with 50% still nursing at 5-6 months postpartum.

The medicinal properties of breastmilk extend not only to the recipient but to the supplier as well. Not only are breastfed babies healthier, but studies show women who nurse receive long-term protection from a number of illnesses, including urinary tract infections, hip fractures, osteoporosis, and breast, cervical, and ovarian cancers. A woman who breastfeeds for two years is significantly less likely to contract breast cancer than a woman who has never lactated.

The potential health and cost savings produced by breastmilk's health advantages have been overlooked by the health, education, government, and business sectors—all of whom stand to benefit if these savings are realized. Unlike many other preventive health measures, breastfeeding costs very little beyond providing proper nutrition, encouragement, and support to breastfeeding mothers. And unlike many preventive measures that can take decades to appreciate savings in health costs, breastfeeding produces cost savings within the first few weeks and months.

Breastfeeding is not difficult or complicated. It is an art, however, and like any art requires study and practice. It takes some effort for mothers and babies to settle into a smooth breastfeeding routine. Most problems women encounter are not medical but are the result of incorrect feeding techniques, lack of information about the art of breastfeeding, ignorance on the part of health care providers, and lack of support from health care workers and family. The answer to breastfeeding problems is seldom to switch to a bottle of formula, but rather to seek out help from someone knowledgeable. Even mothers who have the sense that "breast is best" are subjected to ingrained habits and the expectations of a society that does not embrace breastfeeding as a cultural norm. Unfortunately, successful breastfeeding in this culture often requires determination and confidence and support.

The requirement of determination is the new piece of the equation. The art of breastfeeding hasn't changed since the first cave babies were suckled under fur skins. What's more, the importance of breastmilk in our history is indisputable. Through breastmilk, the human race has remained a viable species on this planet. Without breastmilk, it is highly unlikely that we could have evaded extinction. Infants have survived wars, famine, and concentration camps on nothing but human milk. It is only very recently that a nonbreastfed infant would even be a candidate for survival. Until this century, artificial feeding meant almost certain death.

But many people don't believe that the historical dependence on breastmilk as an infant food makes it necessarily a better choice in today's modern world. After all, clean water is readily available, dishwashers make sterilizing bottles a cinch, and a wide variety of formulas are sold to meet the needs of any infant. Yet, in spite of our modern lifestyles, there remains a connection between the facts that the United States has one of the lowest breastfeeding rates and one of the highest infant mortality rates—in the industrialized world.

Even where bacterial contamination can be minimized, the risks of bottle-feeding are not inconsequential. Bottle-fed infants raised by educated women in clean environments, to this day, have significantly greater rates of illness, hospitalization, and death than breastfed infants. In a study that analyzed hospitalization patterns for a homogeneous, middle-class, white American population, bottle-fed infants were fourteen times more likely to be hospitalized than breastfed infants. Federal health officials have estimated that in 1992, 8,168 deaths occurred as a direct result of the withholding of breastmilk. At current birth-rate levels, over 8,000 families each year are faced with mourning an unnecessary, preventable death.

For many families in this world, progress has meant a significant reduction in, or even the elimination of, breastfeeding. Western ideas, so often viewed as "modern," have altered the attitudes and behaviors of many places on this planet. Advertisers have succeeded in creating the notion that it is mainstream and intelligent to bottle-feed. In many parts of the world, breastfeeding rates have plummeted as women have become more "educated" and affluent. Here in the West, the opposite phenomenon can be seen: the more educated and affluent the woman, the more breastfeeding is a priority. Over 70% of college graduates breastfeed; less than 15% of women with no high school breastfeed (fifty years ago, the opposite was true). Regardless of which groups are studied, the big picture remains the same. With a few notable exceptions (such as Sweden and Australia, where almost all new moms nurse), breastfeeding rates, in America and around the world, are shockingly low.

Infatuation with technology and consumerism has led to the assumption that scientists in sterile laboratories can improve on mother nature. Savvy marketing executives have succeeded in promoting artificial foods as viable "lifestyle alternatives" or "humanized milk," allowing women to be relieved of the burdens of nature through the wonders of modern science. In a world where those things that are "new and improved" are revered, breastfeeding is increasingly eschewed, seen as old, dated, primitive, even unnecessary. That women have been breastfeeding since cave days is viewed as a negative fact rather than as an affirmation of the simplicity and felicitousness of the act. But breastmilk has passed the test of time, and to this day it is compellingly superior to any "new" or "improved" product that can be bought.

Although developed as a medicinal food for sick infants, the profits realized by the manufacturers of formula provided the incentive to transform bottle-feeding into the norm and breastfeeding into the exception. Aggressive advertising, extensive marketing, and cozy relationships with the medical profession have propelled formula into one of the fastest growing and most profitable industries in the world. Florida's Attorney General calculated that for every dollar formula companies charge for wholesale infant formula, the cost of production and delivery is just 16¢. Infant formula sales have comprised up to 50% of the *total* profits of Abbott Laboratories (makers of Similac and Isomil), an enormous pharmaceutical concern. A relentless barrage of advertising and marketing over the decades has embedded our society with the notion that formula-feeding has become so simple, so safe, and so uniformly successful that breastfeeding no longer seems worth the bother.

One of the manifestations of that notion has been the development of "insufficient milk syndrome," a disease that virtually didn't exist years ago and is now being diagnosed more frequently. Women become increasingly convinced that they are incapable of feeding their child, while the fact remains that it is practically unknown for a mammal in her normal environment to produce live young and not be able to suckle them. This is borne out in many traditional societies, where the rate of mothers successfully breastfeeding their young is near 100%.

In "modern" societies, women are sent home with samples of formula, and coupons for more, from the moment the pregnancy is confirmed. Friends, professionals, and books caution them not to be too disappointed if they don't succeed at breastfeeding and emphasize how common it is for a woman not to have enough milk. Mothers are told that nursing will exclude the father and damage the fragile paternal-child bond. Horror stories abound about cracked, bloody nipples and children who bite their mothers. Advertisers reassure pregnant women that formula is the ticket to a free, easy, and happy transition to parenthood. Hospital staff persuade new mothers that formula and sugar water are appropriate for all babies, and stress how much the moms will regret it if they don't get the baby used to a rubber nipple early. Bottle-feeding is so pervasive that in many public facilities, such as international airports and ferry terminals, a baby bottle is used as a symbol to designate these nurseries.

Women who seek counsel from doctors often find them enthusiastic supporters of bottle-feeding. Doctors, nurses, and hospital administrators have collaborated with formula companies for many years and for many reasons. So while it is easy to target the formula companies as the culprits in the battle against breastfeeding, a good amount of the responsibility falls squarely on the shoulders of medical providers. Instead of the medical establishment encouraging women to nurse and giving them the necessary knowledge and support, doctors have spent tremendous time and effort inventing substitute foods that resemble breastmilk, working on ever-better ways to dry up the breasts postpartum, and handing out pamphlets and videos produced by formula companies.

Why are medical providers so quick to promote formula? First and foremost, it is much more profitable. There is much money to be made when an almost free substance is replaced by a costly, inferior one. Hospitals reap millions of dollars awarding exclusive contracts to distribute samples of formula to all maternity patients. And professional medical organizations who endorse bottle feeding, such as the American Association of Pediatricians (AAP), have benefited handsomely from forging cozy relationships with formula companies. Second, encouraging women to use artificial foods allows for synchronization and standardization—which means doctors and nurses can quantify exactly what goes into a baby and dictate when feedings occur. Third, it is much more convenient for nursing staff to give bottles to fussing children than it is to deliver each child to its mother for each feeding. Fourth, doctors have traditionally had very little training in breastfeeding and are often unaware of its benefits and unable to solve the problems of those who experience difficulties. Fifth, artificial foods lead to dramatic weight gain—which makes everyone happy where bigger is considered better. Authors of a 1991 Scandinavian study (Nylander et al., 1991) reviewing hospital procedures surrounding breastfeeding found:

The interference of the medical profession in the twentieth century in the feeding of healthy, term infants may in the future be regarded as a puzzling, uncontrolled, less than well-founded medical experiment.

So rampant is the medical support of bottle-feeding, and so persuasive is the medical case against bottle-feeding, that the Executive Director of UNICEF recently called on all physicians to pledge to do their part to protect, promote and support breastfeeding.

Particularly disturbing is the fact that the abundance of artificial foods and their tacit approval by doctors and hospitals has succeeded in undermining women's confidence in their own ability to produce breastmilk. Almost every woman can provide details about someone who failed trying. Aside from the ramifications the accompanying lack of breastfeeding has on the child's health and the mother's physical health, it also contributes to changes in the mother's mental health. Experts have long known that feeling physically competent is essential to a person's overall self-esteem. Failing at something so basic as feeding one's own child can affect a woman's psyche.

The combination of aggressive advertising, medical backing, and a love of consumer freedom has led to a free-market paradise where a plethora of instant foods are readily available and women have been led to believe that the choice between formula-feeding and breastfeeding is merely a matter of personal inclination—a feather in the cap in the quest for liberation.

In fact, the whole notion of choice is the logic that formula companies use to defend their products. Who wouldn't agree with the concept that rational adults should be able to make their own decisions? After all, America is a country founded on individualism. But the problem with wrapping the "Freedom of Choice" flag around the issues surrounding infant formula is that choice is an illusion unless one is actually presented with accurate information. The choices women are making are based on what has come to be known as "Tainted Truth," the result of extensive advertising and industry-sponsored research. After all, how many of these facts about infant feeding are common knowledge:

- Numerous infants have died or been injured because of formula batches that were incorrectly mixed or contained substances that should not be there. Between 1983 and 1994, the FDA issued twenty-two recalls because of formula safety, over half of which were for problems wherein the product would cause serious health consequences (such as salmonella contamination, broken glass bits, and bacteria that cause sepsis and meningitis).

- Formula-fed infants may be at higher risk for ingesting iodine and aluminum, as well as other heavy metals.

- Formula-fed infants have more learning and behavior difficulties than breastfed infants, and one recent study found that premature infants fed formula have lower IQs. (Lucas)

- Longer chain polyunsaturated fatty acids, which are present in breastmilk but not in formula milks, are vital for brain development. (Lanting 1994, Lucas 1992)

- Formula sales have tripled over the past ten years. The industry is now bigger than ever, generating an astounding $22 million *every day* in revenues—when the superior substance is free! Industry executives know that their products have not even begun to reach market saturation. If every baby in the world were bottle-fed for 6 months, $104 million would be spent on formula every day.

- The U.S. government provides free formula to 37% of all infants born in this country, using over $500 million in tax dollars each year to fund the "gifts."

- Women across the United States have been discriminated against, harassed, even arrested for breastfeeding. The act of breastfeeding is now protected by law in only ten states.

- Women who breastfeed have fewer urinary tract infections; a reduced risk of hip fractures and osteoporosis; and lower rates of breast, cervical, and ovarian cancer.

- The drug, Parlodel, until recently used for lactation suppression, has been responsible for hundreds of serious side effects in new mothers, including seizures, strokes, and heart attacks—at least thirteen of them fatal.

- Breastmilk is one of the few foodstuffs that is packaged and delivered to the consumer without any pollution, unnecessary packaging, or waste. Formula is produced and delivered at significant cost to the environment. If every child in America were bottle-fed, almost 86,000 tons of tin would be needed to produce 550 million cans for just one year's worth of formula. If every mother in the United Kingdom breastfed, 3,000 tons of paper (labels) would be saved in one year. It would take 135 million lactating cows, requiring 43% of the surface of India, to substitute the breastmilk of the women of India.

- The infant formula industry was created not because of problems with breastmilk but because of improvements in mechanization, transportation, and storage, which allowed the dairy industry to thrive. Faced with an increase in waste products, milk processors sought out additional markets. Infant formula was seen as a lucrative outlet for altered waste products from the dairy industry.

- Many medical professionals admit that they withhold breastfeeding information from mothers so the women won't feel guilty if they choose not to do it (women are seen as needing protection from knowing the possible consequences of making a poor choice).

- Breastmilk is assimilated instantly, so breastfeeding mothers can soothe and feed their babies at any time, giving the mother and baby a gentle and even rhythm. Formula takes hours to digest. Formula feedings need to be spaced at no sooner than three-hour intervals, so in-between feedings, pacifiers, and water bottles must be used to try to soothe an unhappy child.

- Health care experts project that if all mothers were to breastfeed for just twelve weeks after giving birth, the United States infant mortality rate (near 89,000 deaths/year) would decline by almost 5%.

Breastfeeding is a bipartisan, pro-health, pro-family, pro-environment issue that saves tax dollars. But there is always a reason not to breastfeed. Some say that human milk is dirty. Grandparents will often tell new mothers that breastfeeding spoils children. The reasons for not breastfeeding shift every few years. For a while, the "in" reason was the concern over "contaminants in mothers' milk." Next was the concern that breastmilk "led to the development of high cholesterol." After that came "breastfeeding is a precursor to sexual abuse." The reasons given for not breastfeeding vary from the misguided ("nursing passes on the mother's allergies") to the inane (self-appointed psychologists insist that the close attachment of a breastfed baby to its mother is at the root of homosexuality).

Two common reasons given today for not breastfeeding are "it excludes the father from participating fully in the care of the baby" and "formula is fine, after all, I wasn't breastfed and I turned out o.k." It is laudable that fathers today are interested in sharing in both the burdens and the joys of raising a child. But sharing is not the same as equivalency. Pregnancy and breastfeeding are things only the mother can do, but that does not mean that there aren't ways for fathers to participate. Anyone who has ever raised a baby can recite all the tasks that need to be done. Babies need holding, stroking, dressing, bathing, comforting, burping, and, within a short time, feeding solids. Dad can do every one of these. The desire to participate should not be confused with the need to give the baby the best of what each partner has to offer.

It is true that formula-fed babies are perfectly capable of growing up into responsible, caring adults. It is also true that many formula-fed adults had repeat bouts of ear infections and diarrhea, needed braces, and still suffer from asthma and allergies. Some studies suggest that adults who were not breastfed have higher rates of heart disease and cancer. In the 1940s and '50s, women typically enjoyed coffee, smoked cigarettes, and drank alcohol during their pregnancies, but this is no longer acceptable. Perhaps as the benefits of breastmilk become better known, there will be recognition that formula-feeding provides for survival, but breastfeeding gives the infant the best start.

Many men and women confuse breastfeeding with obscenity since the breasts are such a key aspect of female sexuality. This issue tends to go away as women gain confidence in, and respect the importance of, breastfeeding. They not only discover that very little of the breast needs to be exposed in order to nurse, but they also alter the image of their own breasts from being sexual organs to being magnificent feeding vessels. One of the best stories about breastfeeding in public comes to us from Wolf Trap Farm Park outside Washington, DC. Women attending an event at the facility were told they could not breastfeed—because nursing attracted bees. When *The Washington Post* ran a story on the incident, park officials confessed that the real reason they had banned breastfeeding was to prevent people from becoming distracted during shows. They then reversed their policy and announced that breastfeeding women were most certainly welcome. When the attitude is taken that a woman's breasts belong to her and no job is more important than caring for one's young, the confusion between breastfeeding and obscenity goes away.

The liberation women need is the ability to breastfeed free of social, medical, and employer constraints. Instead, they have been presented with the notion that liberation comes with being able to abandon breastfeeding without guilt. This "liberation," though, is an illusion representing a distorted view of what breastfeeding is, what breastfeeding does, and what both mothers and babies need after birth. Artificial feeding is giving a child a processed fluid flowing through a piece of rubber. Breastmilk is a living biological fluid that emanates on demand from the breast and is continuously changing to meet the exact needs of both mother and child. Breastfeeding ensures the optimal health and development for the child, while providing the mother with important protection against disease as well.

Breastfeeding is not just the mother giving milk to an open-mouthed baby. A baby has to work for breastmilk by asking for it, then suckling properly to maintain the milk production. It is the baby's suckling and the mother's interaction that keeps the whole process going. The English word "suckle" is so appropriate because it means the action of both the mother and the baby—coworkers. As Gabrielle Palmer explains, "Breastfeeding is really an inadequate word because it is not merely supplying food, it also encompasses bonding and an involvement in an almost magical process. The German word for breastfeeding, *stillen*, means to quieten and soothe rather than to give food." In fact, in some cultures, men may offer their nipple to provide comfort to a crying baby whose mother is absent. Nothing matches breastfeeding as a powerful process for creating closeness. In fact, there are several documented studies that show a noted reduction in the numbers of abandoned babies in societies where breastfeeding rates have risen.

This book is not meant to be a tirade against formula. It is not meant to start a movement to ban artificial foods. It is meant to balance the scales of information, to make informed choice a reality. We believe that all infants would be better off if they were to receive some breastmilk. We also know there is a role for formula in this society. But it is the right of every mother to know the risks to herself and her child if she chooses bottle-feeding over breastfeeding.

This book examines breastfeeding attitudes, customs, and practices of people over time, all around the world—from tribal cultures to high society, from farm families to urban centers. It examines the trends and fashions in breastfeeding, explores why it has been the focus of so much attention, and looks at how the search for alternative foods sheds light on just how miraculous breastmilk really is. It also shows how easily breastfeeding is eroded. It is not a how-to book, but rather is designed to serve as a companion resource to any of the many excellent how-to books available. Each chapter presents different material and is meant to stand on its own. A number of appendices are provided to supply additional information.

In order to reduce the downward trend in breastfeeding, governments, nongovernmental groups, and international health agencies are working together in a concerted effort to promote, support, and protect breastfeeding. Spurred by UNICEF, efforts are underway to put an end to free and low-cost supplies of infant formula. It is our hope that through this book it will become clear that breastfeeding is not only a woman's right and an infant's best start, but that it can also be a delightful experience for both mother and baby that is as beneficial physically as it is emotionally.

Section I

Breastfeeding Beliefs and Practices

One

Breastfeeding Customs around the World

The reproduction of the species—their nurture in the womb, and their support and culture during infancy and childhood—is the grand prerogative of woman. It is a noble and a holy office, to which she is appointed by God, and the duty is both pure and sacred.
—William H. Cook, *Woman's Hand-Book of Health*, 1866

People like to believe that mothering is instinctual, a skill, unleashed by hormones, possessed by every female. That is simply not true. Both men and women must learn how to nurture. Each society establishes its own approaches and guidelines for how each gender should tend to the needs of the young. Breastfeeding, that most ancient of feeding methods, is an integral part of mothering, and it, too, is a learned art (Figure 1.1). Just because the breasts fill with milk upon the birth of a child does not mean that breastfeeding occurs easily and universally. How it is done, how often, and by whom varies within communities and among generations.

The study of nonhuman primates has shown that attitudes toward both sex and suckling are established early in life by the young closely watching the adults. If chimpanzees, for instance, are deprived of this exposure, they develop problems with both activities when they reach maturity. Likewise, mothering does not occur in a vacuum but is part of a continuum of human life where the mother and her newborn infant are woven into each society's fabric of family structure and community life.

This chapter explores maternal customs and practices around the world. It examines how different cultures experience motherhood and looks at attitudes and breastfeeding practices in the mothering process. Birth and motherhood are universal experiences, but individual experiences of being pregnant, giving birth, and entering motherhood vary widely.

Figure 1.1
Playing Mom

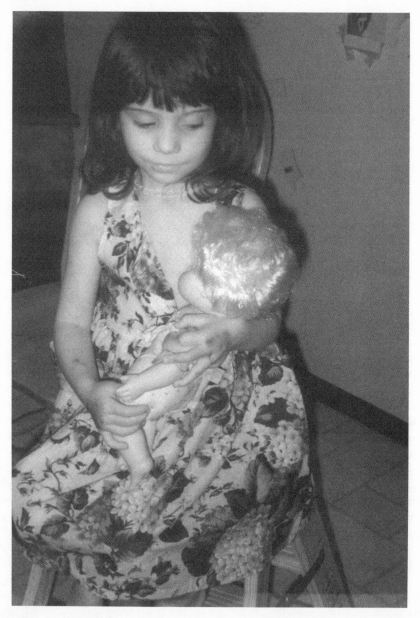

This four-year-old mimics her mother by "breastfeeding" her doll, but most children do not know about breastfeeding and only have experience with bottle-feeding. When a little boy played at breastfeeding in one Montessori nursery school, the teacher labeled it as aberrant behavior. *Photo courtesy*: Dia L. Michels.

There are strong religious messages for women to be both fertile and maternal. Among the Yoruba of West Nigeria, the goddess of fertility is Odudua, depicted as a woman nursing twins. In ancient Egypt, one of the mother-goddesses was Bast, represented by a cat nursing kittens. In Aztec culture, infants dying while still being nursed went to a special afterlife. Talmudic law prescribes that Jewish babies be breastfed at least twenty-four months. In the Old Testament, the most severe punishment for the erring Israelites was for God to give them a miscarrying womb and a dry breast. The Bible tells us that nursing her babies is a mother's sacred duty that should take precedence over all other obligations. Lactating breasts are considered God's blessing; a mother who neglects her infant is compared to the ostrich ("daughter of greediness"), a bird that deserts her eggs in the desert to hatch by themselves.

Regardless of the strong religious direction to breastfeed, infant feeding fashions run in cycles. While there are increases in the breastfeeding rates at certain times among certain groups, the overall pattern, both in the United States and around the world, is one of increased reliance on artificial feeding.

Even though breastfeeding has long been the passport to infant survival, prejudice against breastfeeding has always existed. The justifications for the prejudice vary, but there has never been a time when notable people didn't consider breastfeeding either disgusting, unwomanly, or unhealthy. A disdain for breastfeeding has long been evident among the wealthiest classes. As far back as biblical times, fashionable women were unwilling to nurse their own children. The Bible tells us that these women were chided by Jeremiah: "Even the sea monsters draw out the breast. They give suck to their young."

A passage in the book *Abyss*, published in 1903, gives us the following observation:

In a narrow doorway, so narrow that perforce we stepped over her, sat a woman with a young babe, nursing at breasts grossly naked and libeling all the sacredness of motherhood. (Jack London, *Abyss*, 1903)

This passage is but one example of the distaste for breastfeeding long held by the upper class.

It would be nice to dismiss the long-standing upper-class derision of breastfeeding as foolishness affecting just a small percentage of the population, but upper-class preferences historically have had significant influence on the attitudes toward breastfeeding throughout the whole society. Emulation of the rich occurs in every culture. The more the upper classes have focused on the breasts as decorative and the less accessible they are in the fashions of the time, the more interest there has been in finding alternative means of feeding babies.

In Europe, until the fifteenth century, women's clothing was loose and relatively comfortable, and breastfeeding was the norm, even for noblewomen. But by the sixteenth century, fashion had taken on a new significance for upper-class women. A woman's body was viewed more as an object of decoration than as an object of utility. Clothing that made work impossible helped to define the status of upper-class women as members of the society who did not work. Fashionable women were donning corsets of leather, bone, or even metal to give shape to high-necked garments that fastened in the back. Not only did these fashions make access to the breasts impossible, but some garments so severely flattened the breasts and nipples that they actually damaged the internal organs and, in some cases, cracked ribs. Chinese upper-class women who wore very tight and completely flattening dresses were unable to breastfeed.

The rich have not held a monopoly on negative attitudes toward breastfeeding, but of course they most often have had the means to search for alternatives.

BREASTS AS SEX SYMBOLS

The dictionary defines *breast* as "either of two milk-secreting glands protruding from the upper, front part of a woman's body." Traditionally, breasts have been considered organs of lactation and have been exposed without inhibition. As cultures have become "civilized," breasts have been transformed from functional items to objects of female decoration and sexual organs whose purpose in life is to titillate and stimulate. As our preoccupation with the breasts as tools for sexual stimulation has increased, there has been a corresponding reduction in usage for their primary lactating function. Our culture, proud of its high standards of morality and modernization (and abetted by advertising images of the body beautiful), has transformed the breast into a sexual, from a sustenance, object. The image of a woman walking around with an exposed breast (no matter that a suckling infant is attached to it) has been wrongly equated with a man walking around with his penis hanging out. It is this attitude that leads to situations such as the one where a woman was harassed by a security guard for nursing her child in a Florida shopping mall in 1992 and the incident in St. Louis in 1981, where a mother who was quietly nursing her infant in her parked car was warned that she was indecently exposed. Breastfeeding is so rare in U.S. culture that there are many such incidents nationwide of women being harassed while breastfeeding by security guards, shop assistants, swimming pool club members, and ignorant onlookers. No mother has been formally arrested or cited for breastfeeding. Most mothers are told to leave the establishment. Some do and some don't. New laws are being added in many states to "clarify" what we already know—that breastfeeding is not criminal behavior (Appendix G).

In societies where there is no shame attached to breastfeeding, the ordinary man is not driven into a frenzy by the mere sight of a female breast. Until recently, women have been able to feed babies in even the most sexually repressive societies, feeding comfortably in public even in places where women do not customarily show their faces. In Victorian England, known for its views of sexual propriety, a respectable woman would think nothing of feeding openly even in church.

In developing countries, women don't think twice about being nursing mothers with bare breasts exposed, but in so-called developed countries, the teleologic use of the breasts causes derision and embarrassment. For instance, when a class of third graders in Cincinnati, Ohio, viewed a cultural film on the Kalahari Bush people, they were more concerned with the sight of the Bush women's breasts than with their lifestyle. When women start feeling self-conscious about exposure of their breasts, they start thinking about other ways to feed their infants.

Women are bombarded today by images of "the ideal woman," with messages that love, acceptance, and approval from men are dependent on the right appearance. The right appearance, in this case, involves the right size breasts as an essential part of female decoration. What is fashionable in breast size varies (in the Roaring Twenties, flat chests were the rage), but the notion that perfectly formed breasts are crucial to a happy life is pervasive today throughout our culture. A memo in the early 1980s to the Food and Drug Administration (FDA) from the American Society of Plastic and Reconstructive Surgeons stated:

There is a substantial and enlarging body of medical information and opinion to the effect that these deformities [small breasts] are really a disease [that left uncorrected, results in a] total lack of well being.

Among the most popular "cures" for this "disease" has been silicone-gel breast implants touted as being a simple and minor surgical procedure. Over two million American women have spent thousands of dollars, eliminated their option to breastfeed, and put themselves at significant medical risk in order to have their breasts surgically "enhanced." In 1990 alone, 130,000 American women had their breasts augmented, a business generating $450 million annually for the coffers of plastic surgeons. Federal regulators at the FDA have stood idly by in spite of mounting reports on the frightening, and sometimes fatal, health consequences of these implants. The more value a society places on women for their role as sexual beings, the more women shun exposure of and utility from their breasts. The more women total their self-worth as the sum of their body parts, the more they are willing to endanger their health and their children's health in pursuit of an image.

INTERCOURSE TABOOS

Many cultures prohibit sexual intercourse during pregnancy and for the period of time the mother is lactating. The stated reasons for the prohibitions vary, but all are based on the desire to protect the child. Current western medicine does not seek to limit or reduce intercourse during normal pregnancies and only restricts coital relations for a few weeks postpartum. Traditional taboos calling for intercourse restrictions, however, may have been more than quaint folklore. There is some evidence that, among malnourished women, intercourse late in pregnancy can lead to an increased number of uterine infections and premature births.

Taboos limiting sexual relations postpartum are rooted in age-old wisdom. In addition to allowing the new mother more time with, and energy for, her child, an intercourse taboo serves the very practical purpose of postponing future pregnancies. Mothers who breastfeed exclusively (that is, frequently, on demand, including during the night, with no supplementation) generally enjoy a period of natural birth control. One study of Senegalese women documented that a breastfeeding duration of 22.8 months produced a postpartum lactation infertility period of 18.2 months. This natural means of birth control is lost when breastfeeding is reduced (as in formula supplementation) or when the child is weaned. In Zaire, it was found that only 5% of mothers breastfeeding their 12–18 month old infants were pregnant, as compared to 60% of nonbreastfeeding mothers. In many cultures, breastfeeding is prolonged for two or more years, and during this entire period intercourse is taboo.

It is a fact that, in developing countries, children born less than two years after their next older sibling are almost twice as likely to die as those born more than two years apart. Spacing is considered one of the most important contributors to infant death. Intercourse taboos combined with the natural contraceptive effects of nursing prevent huge numbers of infant deaths as well as a considerable amount of maternal mortality as well. Where food shortages are common, disease endemic, and survival difficult, a mother can barely feed herself and her infant, let alone another infant in the womb.

Bodily fluids come with a wide array of folklore and breastmilk is no different. Many cultures believe that semen will curdle, or even poison, the breastmilk. Zulu tradition claims that manhood may be lost if breastmilk falls on a man's skin. Such customs are still observed in many areas of the world. Intercourse taboos are better respected where polygamy exists, but, of course, most of the world no longer condones such arrangements. Even in cultures where intercourse and breastfeeding can be mixed, the latter still affords some protection against future pregnancies.

Now that artificial foods are widely available, even in remote regions, some husbands are pressuring their wives to switch to artificial feeding as a way of circumventing the intercourse taboo. Migrant workers in Lesotho, for example, who returned from working in the mines, bought their wives cans of formula as formula-feeding allowed them to bypass the taboo. Hard-earned currency then goes to the formula companies, while the woman is more likely to find herself with a sick child and another pregnancy.

In every culture, there is an increased morbidity when nursing ceases early. In cultures where survival is difficult, the continuation of breastfeeding is a life-and-death issue. Yet in many societies a new pregnancy almost results in an abrupt halt to nursing. Mothers, and even doctors, fear that breastfeeding could not only harm the infant at the breast but also the infant in utero. The Zulus believe that a new baby in the womb is rightful owner of the milk and that, if the nursing mother becomes pregnant, the existing baby's milk supply will be contaminated, harming the nursing child. In the event of a new pregnancy, the infant is immediately taken off the breast and sent to the grandmother, or a noxious substance, such as bitter herb, aloe, pepper, or iodine, is applied to the breasts to discourage suckling. As there is no available dietary substitute for breastmilk in many poor societies, a new pregnancy often spells disaster for the nursing child. Hence, the longer the interval between births, the better.

Aside from issues of survival in third-world nations, breastfeeding and pregnancy can be perfectly compatible. Breastfeeding one baby while growing another can be taxing for the mother, but a well-nourished woman can continue to breastfeed while pregnant without fetus, child, or mother suffering any harmful effects. Even though there is nothing that precludes breastfeeding during pregnancy, Mother Nature does a bit of adjusting. When a lactating woman becomes pregnant, hormonal changes occur and the milk composition begins to change. The mature milk slowly begins to reverse, first back to immature milk, then to colostrum. Colostrum tastes different from mature milk, and because it is thick and sticky it does not flow freely. Older nursing infants often comment on the sour taste of the milk, and mothers have noticed these children develop "lactation diarrhea," probably due to the laxative effect of colostrum. At the same time that the amount of milk is diminishing and the taste is worsening, the mother's nipples become more tender. The breast swelling and nipple pain that often accompany pregnancy still accompany pregnancy when lactating. It seems this is a natural method of weaning in preparation for the new baby in that the mother's pleasure in providing the breastmilk diminishes at the same time that the child's pleasure in receiving the milk is reduced.

"Progress" threatens breastfeeding in more ways than through the availability of artificial foods. Child spacing achieved by the artificial means of birth control is a relatively new phenomena. Oral contraceptives, often resumed shortly after an infant is delivered, can be especially harmful to breastfeeding, as estrogen is known to reduce the flow of breastmilk. Plus, when infants are born in hospitals, women from traditional cultures may discard some very good traditions. For example, in Swaziland, Zululand, Lesotho, and Malawi, traditional women are considered "unclean" after delivery and sexual intercourse is taboo. The face and hands of lactating women in some African tribes are painted white with a special clay designating them as untouchable. Among the Niger nomads, a lactating woman has to wear special beads (Figure 1.2). But nowadays, more and more women are delivering in hospitals and women who have hospital births are regarded as "cleaned out" and in some societies the taboo against intercourse is dropped. Changes of this type result in closer child spacing, an increase in infant malnutrition, and an increase in child mortality.

Not only does breastfeeding provide a natural means of birth control, but also researchers record that breastfeeding mothers do not resume "normal" sexual relations as quickly as bottle-feeding mothers. The hormone oxytocin, secreted into the woman's body through the process of breastfeeding, helps a nursing mother feel calm and nurturing. It is her body's way of helping her establish a warm loving relationship with her new baby. Her energies are focused on attending to the child and the home. In addition hormones also may lower the level of vaginal lubrication, making sex uncomfortable. Women with lower levels of oxytocin (such as those who don't breastfeed) are more likely to resent the child for being in the way when the parents want to have sex.

The problem is that there is no similar hormonal change in men and this creates a potential area of conflict—men may still want intercourse with the same frequency to which they were accustomed. For men who are not adaptable to the changes in the relationship or do not appreciate the changes a new baby brings to a household, this imbalance can lead to marital conflict and resentment. Unfortunately, women are often instructed to make time for their husbands and to "service" them, if need be, in order to retain marital harmony. Men who have a difficult time adjusting to the wife's sudden shift of time and attention away from the husband, and to the baby, can make life difficult.

It is hard to breastfeed without the support of the spouse. Some women give up nursing so their husbands don't feel threatened. Others continue to nurse, but feel that they do so in spite of their husbands. Many western women have commented that they would welcome an intercourse taboo in the first few months of motherhood.

Figure 1.2
Nursing Mothers Necklace

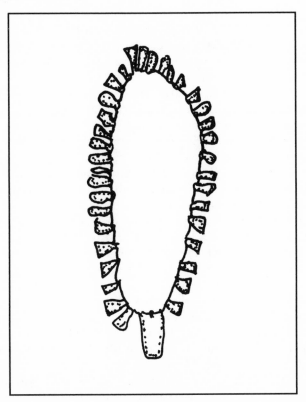

In Niger, nomad nursing mothers wear long leather necklaces to protect them from men and guarantee the growth of their children. As long as a woman wears it, she may not have sexual relations. Only at the end of the child's second year can she remove the necklace, resuming accession to wifehood and marital intercourse. *Drawing Courtesy*: N. Baumslag.

DIET DURING AND AFTER PREGNANCY

All societies have developed their own folklore on what to feed women when they are "with child" or caring for their newborn. During pregnancy, and particularly in the nursing period, it is not uncommon for mothers to be told that harm will come to their babies if they eat certain foods. Specific foods are restricted, others are included and considered special "strength-ening" foods. The differences in diet among cultures reflects differences in attitudes, beliefs, and environmental conditions. From a medical point of view, some of the dietary restrictions make no sense at all, while others may be beneficial for the baby and/or mother. Ironically, many of the foods restricted from the diets of women in developing countries are highly rec-ommended to mothers in the United States.

The extent of these beliefs varies from region to region. Eggs are not eaten by mothers in one area of Tunis, while as many as six to eight eggs a day are eaten in another region. In some African areas, fruit, milk, meat, fish, and eggs are taboo during pregnancy, and the only foods eaten are watered-down local staples such as maize, rice, sour porridge (fermented maize), or bread. These practices are often founded in age-old fears that some foods are responsible for inducing abortions or for bringing harm to mother or fetus. For example, in Sierra Leone, it is believed that if the mother eats fish, the baby will get worms, or if eggs are eaten during preg-nancy, the baby may have a large head or dribble or have convulsions or even grow up to be a thief. In Oman, it is believed that the unborn child is located in the mother's stomach, and that as the fetus grows more space must be left and less food eaten. Mothers in this region also believe that if they eat fish bones and scales, the bones of their fetus will harden and lead to a difficult delivery. Many believe that pregnancy alters digestion, so nu-tritious foods such as beans and lentils are avoided.

In Ethiopia, large amounts of butter are added to the mother's maize por-ridge, and she is often secluded for two months, during which time all her do-mestic chores, including food preparation, are performed by relatives. Desert Bedouin women of the Negev were not allowed to cook for a period of time after a birth. Women of the family gave the new mother meat, eggs, and milk—but only if the husband approves! The wife will be well fed if a son is born. Should the baby die while suckled, the mother's breastmilk is blamed. In addition to being given special foods, Tanzanian mothers also get a two-month resting period. One Tanzanian tribe, the Watching, provides mothers with a diet rich in milk, blood, and fat. If the baby does not thrive, the milk is tested by placing a drop of milk on a plate, and if a fly settles on it, the breastmilk is blamed for the infant's condition. Among some Kenyan tribes, when an infant has died while being breastfed, a mother must have her breasts ritually purified before she can nurse again.

Among many sects in India, after childbirth the mother is allowed cooked rice, bread, and coffee. Vegetables and fish are prohibited, as she is consid-ered unable to digest food. Nor is she allowed to cook; this situation pre-vails in many peasant societies. Muslim women in Bangladesh may not eat animal fat after an infant is born. The mother is considered "polluted" for forty days after the birth, and if the infant falls ill the mother is blamed. Fish is excluded from the diet of Afghanistanee women; it is believed that it interferes with breastfeeding and causes early onset of menstruation. In Sri Lanka, mothers are forbidden to drink cow's milk when nursing. These mothers often obtain much-needed calcium from chewing betel nuts steeped in lime; the betel nuts probably also help improve the let-down reflex. In one East African tribe, new mothers are required to avoid eating chicken; it is thought to cause convulsions and fever in infants. This restriction may limit the mother's protein and iron intake. Common taboos also extend to fruits such as mango, papaya, and coconut, which are thought to reduce the mother's milk production and cause diarrhea.

Some dietary practices are harmful while others are beneficial. In Sierra Leone, pregnant women may not consume any alcohol and, of course, this practice, which has been around for a long time, is sound. Only recently have western scientists come to realize the danger to the baby when the expectant mother drinks alcohol (babies may be born with facial abnormalities, retarded growth, or serious mental defects). Among the Somalis, pregnant women are encouraged to eat liver, a food high in Vitamins A, B12, and iron. These nutrients are important for blood formation, and restricted diets are frequently short of these essential blood-forming factors. Anemia in pregnancy and in infancy is very common all over the world and is usually caused by iron deficiency, *however*, folic acid deficiency is also not an uncommon cause of anemia. Dietary restrictions during lactation can also be beneficial; for instance, cow's milk and coconut, commonly off limits to nursing mothers, often provoke allergic reactions in infants.

CRAVINGS IN PREGNANCY

It is common knowledge that pregnant women often have peculiar cravings for foods such as pickles or chocolates. Pregnancy cravings were well known and described even in fairy tales. In *Rapunzel,* the mother became pale and weak (which are signs of nutritional anemia), so the father stole rampunion to treat her. Centuries later, scientists discovered that greens like rampunion are high in folic acid and that a deficiency of this substance causes a form of pregnancy anemia. Common thought has long held that women crave substances that provide them with nutrients that are lacking in the diet, but it took a long time before researchers established a scientific basis for some of these cravings. Many are however still unexplained.

Cravings during pregnancy are commonplace. And cravings aren't necessarily even for foodstuffs. Obsessive-compulsive eating of nonfoodstuffs is known as *pica,* which means "magpie" (magpies are known to eat anything). Some pregnant women eat twigs, paper, ashes, dirt, and ice, to name a few items.

The most common of the nonfoods compulsively eaten is clay or earth (known as *geophagia,* or earth-eating). In the third century BC, Plato noticed pregnant Greek women snacking on dirt. This practice of eating earth is widespread and found all over the world from the United States to Africa. In Sierra Leone, it is called *dotti*. Women who crave earth go to extraordinary lengths to obtain it.

Cravings for clay are well-known in the United States. The practice among American black women is believed to have originated in Africa and traveled here with the slaves. Today, clay eating is considered a disgusting habit, yet it was not always thought so. In Roman times, clay was sold in pills and prescribed as medicine. Clay, packaged especially for pregnant women, can be found in villages and cities around the globe. It has been desired from Kinchassa, Zaire, to Atlanta, Georgia. Pregnant women in Cincinnati used to obtain clay from Georgia. Clay was sold regularly at markets in Atlanta until the health department banned it. Banning it did not eliminate the desire, it simply forced the product underground, making supervision and monitoring more difficult. Clay is also used by traditional healers for dysentery and gastrointestinal complaints. Clay contains kaolite, which is the active ingredient in the anti-diarrhea preparation Kaopectate. The anti-diarrheal effect may be but one reason for geophagia.

There are several forms that pica takes in pregnancy. One is ash eating, which was a well-known form of pica even in Eastern Europe. Another item sought after compulsively during pregnancy is ice; cravings for ice are called *pagophagia*. Some women have been known to eat as many as five trays of ice a day, in some cases, even scraping the frost off the refrigerator coils. Other forms of pica include the craving for special brands of laundry starch, called *amylophagia*. It has been suggested that some starch eaters have switched from earth to starch because the product looks cleaner, has a better taste, and is easier to purchase in urban areas. Eating starch, though, may pose greater health hazards than eating earth.

There are a number of studies that suggest that pica in pregnancy is frequently associated with anemia and the cravings tend to disappear when the anemia is treated and iron levels are raised. Still, the exact cause of pica remains a mystery.

THE FEAR OF LABOR AND DELIVERY

Women, universally, fear a difficult labor and delivery. Those who deliver in the bush, at home, or alone far from health services have good reason to fear. They know, and fear, the risks of infant and maternal death in childbirth. The well-founded fear of giving birth to a large baby is especially great, particularly in places with no obstetrical services when women have contracted pelvises. Such pelvic distortion can result from rickets, a disease caused by lack of sunlight and/or Vitamin D, calcium, or potassium. Rickets has been found in Glasgow among slum dwellers and as far afield as in Bedouins of the Negev desert, where women are covered in cloth and confined to tents or shelters and do not get exposed to sunlight.

As late as the early twentieth century, rickety contracted pelvises were still a problem in Germany. Operating under the belief (for which minimal proof exists) that a smaller baby would lead to an easier delivery, a German doctor named Prochownik drastically reduced the caloric intake of women with small or contracted pelvises. His patients did have easier labors—at the expense of delivering pitifully small infants, many of whom died. Dietary restrictions still exist in a number of cultures. The Masai women of Kenya, who normally eat a diet on which any fetus would thrive, subsist largely on watered-down porridge during pregnancy in an effort to minimize fetal size. Small, frail, sickly babies often result. Sadly, their customary foods, high in protein (including meat, milk, and fresh cattle blood), are taboo during pregnancy.

Only in recent years have American women been instructed not to restrict pregnancy weight gain. Limiting the amount of weight one gained was thought to reduce the chances of developing pregnancy toxemia. In the 1930s, fifteen pounds was the recommended maximum weight gain. In the '60s and '70s, the acceptable suggested range rose to 20–25 pounds. Contemporary medical thought has since rejected restrictive caloric regimes, as it has not been shown to reduce the incidence of toxemia but has been shown to increase the incidence of low birth weight infants (who have higher rates of mortality, mental retardation, and other developmental problems). Today, doctors will tell a normal-size woman that she should gain no more than 35 pounds. However, weight is often rigidly monitored and women are instructed to restrict their caloric intake.

American women, in the Baby Boom period after World War II, had extraordinarily low breastfeeding rates. Women were actively discouraged from trying to breastfeed, and those who did were chastised. Doctors bent on the scientific miracle of artificial foods declared breastfed children inadequately nourished and prescribed formula supplementation. Undoubtedly, a number of factors were at play, but one had to be the restricted diets during pregnancy and in the postnatal period. It has been shown that mothers who limited their pregnancy diet had difficulty sustaining their milk supply for three months or more. As field workers have always been aware, if you want to help feed the babies—feed the mothers.

CHILDBIRTH ASSISTANCE

The assumption that a woman and her baby will survive labor and delivery is one that only a percentage of women in this world can make. In many developing countries, procedures, equipment, and resources that save lives are often not available. Many a healthy child has come into this world through an unassisted birth—the Bush women go off on their own—but generally women do have some form of help. Mothers, grandmothers, and extended family assume the role of birth attendants in rural areas.

These Traditional Birth Attendants (TBAs), a term coined by the World Health Organization (WHO), preside over village births and are assisted by younger women apprentices. In much of the world, midwives are the obvious attendants at a birth—doctors are thought of as attendants to sick people. TBAs are and always have been invaluable. They are found in Africa, Latin America, India, Southeast Asia, and numerous Islamic cultures. In Southern Africa, they are called *songomas*; in Indonesia, *dukuns*; in Mexico, *comadronas*; and in the Sudan, they are known as *dias*. In many countries, there are programs to upgrade the skills and practices of illiterate birth attendants. In countries like Sierra Leone, Malawi, and the Sudan, the attendants are taught to recognize emergencies and identify mothers requiring special care. They are taught how and whom to send to hospital, as well as techniques for preventing prolonged labor and minimizing infection.

Birth attendants play a big role in getting the mother off to a good start. These women "mother the mother." They teach them how to take care of themselves in pregnancy, give them massage, help them through delivery, and instruct them on caring for the newborn. They assist mothers with breastfeeding, and some even see that the children are taken to clinics for their shots. Such attention after the birth is fundamental to promoting breastfeeding and warding off potential disasters.

In our own "advanced" health system, the trained and certified midwife is often prevented from performing home births and offering any services other than prenatal checkups and supervising hospital deliveries with a doctor in attendance. Instead of allowing midwives to provide alternate choices and backup services to the community, doctors block midwives from practicing—and thus competing—except in those areas where doctors don't want to work (such as among the rural poor, where there is an obstetrical shortage). Generally speaking, doctors believe that births should be handled exclusively by doctors in hospitals. This attitude persists despite evidence that midwives (both for hospital and home births) have lower rates of cesarean sections, fewer complications, and cost less than their doctor counterparts.

MOTHERING THE MOTHER

In traditional societies, the time after birth is a period when both mother and baby are given special care. These mothers often have only to feed the baby; family members or attendants are there to care for the home and the child, and to bring the infant to the mother when hungry or when the mother's breasts are full. A true two-way demand feeding is established. During this important initial period, rituals may be performed to keep away evil spirits, and visitors (sometimes including husbands) are excluded.

This is a time for mothers to bond with their infants. It is called a variety of names such as the *lying-in-period, the period of pollution, convalescent period, unclean period,* and *period of confinement.* During this time, which in various cultures lasts from forty days to one year, the mother receives foods intended to increase her strength and promote milk production. She is allowed time for rest and given practical support and advice. She may receive prescribed herbal remedies for "strength," or for "poor" or "low" blood (anemia) both during and after pregnancy; attendance at and help with the delivery; postnatal care; massage; help with care for older children; help with household chores; emotional support; and help with taking care of the new baby.

In parts of South Africa, such as among the Tswana people, the afterbirth as well as hair from the mother, nail clippings, and perhaps a sample of milk are buried in a secret place by an old woman. In China, in the rural areas, as in many developing countries, mother and infant are kept inside for fifty-six days and doors and windows kept closed (not surprisingly, rickets, from lack of sunlight, develops in many of these infants). The mother is not allowed to do housework, sew, read, or cook; the family does all the chores, freeing mom to concentrate on the infant. Considering the high probability of infant mortality, isolation of infant and mother may prevent exposure to infectious diseases at a very vulnerable time.

An entirely different situation exists in societies where technology is emphasized. The birth process is seen from a clinical viewpoint, with obstetricians emphasizing technology. A battery of defensive practices are employed, some of which are totally irrelevant to the health of either mother or infant. Skilled technicians spend their time and the family's money on identifying the baby's gender and performing various stress tests. All the focus is geared toward the actual birth. After the birth, the mother and infant become medically separated. The infant is relegated to the care of the pediatrician, the uterus to the obstetrician, the breast abscess to the surgeon. While the various anatomical parts are given the required care, the person who is the new mother is often left to fend for herself. She is generally given little more than a book or pamphlet, a pep talk, a demonstration here or there, and perhaps a warning that her hormones will be unstable for a while. She is rushed out of the hospital within a day or two of delivery in order to satisfy the requirements of her insurance company (or, if she doesn't have insurance, she is rushed home to free up the bed). All the tender loving care flows to the infant; the mother becomes the unpaid nursemaid.

This may appear to be a harsh evaluation, but it is realistic. In western society, the baby gets attention while the mother is given lectures. Pregnancy is considered an illness; once the "illness" is over, interest in her wanes. Mothers in "civilized" countries often have no or very little help with a new baby. Women tend to be home alone to fend for themselves and the children. They are typically isolated socially and expected to complete their usual chores, including keeping the house clean and doing the cooking and shopping, while being the sole person to care for the infant. Living in sprawling bedroom communities, with two-career couples as neighbors, a car is often required just to find a friendly face.

Women who choose or need to go back to a job after giving birth often must return sooner than they would like to or feel ready to. The lack of governmental policies on maternity leave (and the lack of pay even when such leave is available) means a new mother has to concentrate on preparing to leave the infant at a time when she should be focusing on bonding.

The financial realities of living in today's world, the isolation inherent in modern living arrangements, the lack of paternity leave, and the absence of nearby family can leave the new mother feeling exhausted, overwhelmed, and alone. According to the U.S. rules and regulations governing the federal worker, the pregnancy and postdelivery period is referred to as "the period of incapacitation." This reflects the reality of a situation that should be called "the period of joy." Historically, mothering was a group process with chores and child-minding shared by the available adults. This provided not only needed relief but also readily available advice and experience. Of the "traditional" and "modern" child-rearing situations, it is the modern isolated western mom who is much more likely to find herself experiencing lactation failure.

GALACTOGOGUES

Over the centuries, a wide variety of practices has developed to optimize a safe and sufficient supply of breastmilk. Beliefs and practices designed to promote abundant milk have included prayers, rituals, sexual abstinence, dietary modifications, and medicines for women to take when pregnant and/or lactating. Prayers have been especially prevalent. A particularly good visual example of this is a pair of votive paintings found in Japanese temples (Figure 1.3). One painting depicts a woman praying for a plentiful milk supply; the adjoining painting shows her prayers answered. Women were not the only ones praying for breastmilk. Priests also sought help from above for abundant, flowing milk. According to ancient Jewish sources, it used to be that on Thursdays priests prayed and fasted for nursing mothers to be able to breastfeed their infants.

Some of the remedies proposed are spiritual; many are also herbal and food related. It has long been observed that certain foods affect the production and supply of breastmilk. Some have been found to have a scientific

Figure 1.3
Praying for an Abundant Milk Supply

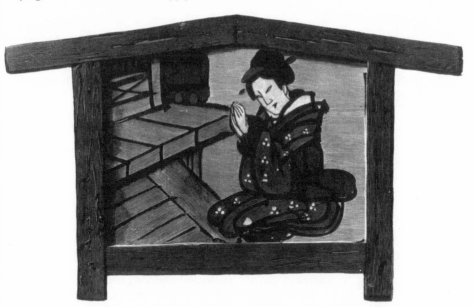

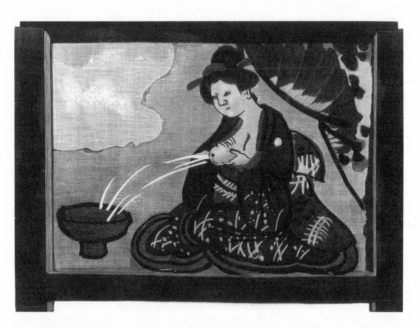

Votive paintings, depicting a mother praying for an abundant milk supply for her newborn infant and her prayer being answered, were found in Japanese temples. *Source*: H.H. Ploss, M. Bartels, and P. Bartels, *Das Weib in der Natur und Volkerkunde: Anthropologische Studien*. 1st ed. (Leipzig: Grieben, 1885). *Photo courtesy*: History of Medicine Division, National Library of Medicine, Bethesda, Maryland.

Table 1.1
Galactogogues

These galactogogues may improve the mother's diet and fluid content, or may reduce anxiety and encourage the let-down reflex. Folklore abounds in regimes to ensure a sufficient milk supply. The following is a partial list of some of the common ingredients in galactogogues.	
India	ginger, jaggery, powdered earthworms
Pakistan	cumin, lassi, cottonseed, goat's stomach
Mexico	gruels made from legumes, ground nuts, chickpeas, sesame seed, cottonseed, absinthe
Tunisia	herb teas called "verveine" made from fennel, coriander seeds, barley, and couscous
United States	milk tea made with thistle, comfrey, and fennel
China	soup made from pigs' hooves, tailbones, and fish tails, boiled with ginger, or cooked with beans and peanuts; eggs; chicken soup made from adult roosters
Nepal	juana seed, fennel, dill, caraway, mustard greens
Guatemala	Ixbut tea from leaves of euphorbia lancifolia plant
Honduras	velvet-bean cocoa drink

Note: These galactogogues have not been subjected to scientific testing. Herbs are a common ingredient in many of these galactogogues. Some may be harmful if taken in megadoses. Recently, comfrey has been found to cause liver damage and blood clots. The use of comfrey leaves has been banned in Canada and Germany. These teas should not be consumed in large amounts. If the constituents of the tea are known, regional poison centers can provide information on the safety of active principles.

basis, while others appear to be little more than popular folklore (which doesn't mean they don't work!). Foods and herbs that increase milk flow are known as galactogogues. Each culture has developed a collection of milk-producing (referred to as galactogenic) substances to help ensure an abundant milk supply or to rectify a milk insufficiency. Galactogogues vary widely (Table 1.1); some Indian tribes swear by powdered earthworm soup, while velvet-bean drinks are popular in Honduras. In western societies, peanuts and Coca Cola are advocated by some doctors, deplored by others. Whatever else peanuts and coke do, they certainly increase calories, fat, and fluid intake. Some galactogogues are geared toward improving and increasing the mother's caloric intake and/or nutritional composition, while others are designed to promote relaxation and thus reduce anxiety and encourage the let-down reflex.

The medical literature abounds in treatments for lactation failure. The *Papyrus Ebers* (1550 BC), the earliest medical encyclopedia, offers a short prescription for the promotion of breastfeeding:

To get a supply of milk in a woman's breasts for suckling the child; warm the bones of a swordfish in oil and rub her back with it. Or, let the woman sit cross-legged and eat fragrant bread of soused durra while rubbing her parts with the poppy plant.

In the sixteenth century, Phayer, a physician, recommended the following in his *Remedie appropriate to ye encreasing of Mylke the Brestes*:

Parsneppe rootes, fenelle roots sodden in broth of chicken and afterwards eaten with a little freshe butter rice soaked in cows milk, powder of earthworms dry and dronken in the broth of a neates tongue, the broth of an old cocke, with myntes, cynanon and maces.

If all this failed, local application of fennel plasters to the breasts was advocated. Arm exercises were also recommended.

The desire to treat lactation failure is as alive today as it was for ancient peoples (Figure 1.4). In Pakistan, galactogogues include cumin, lassi, and cottonseed as well as dried, powdered, goat's stomach. In India, fried ginger, jaggery, black pepper, and ware may be given as a tonic for ten to thirty days. Some remedies from Mexico include atoles (gruels) made from legumes, ground nuts, or chickpeas. Northern Mexicans make teas from so-called "hot plants"—sesame, absinthe, and cottonseed. In other parts of Latin America, herb teas are consumed in the evening to stimulate milk for the next morning. In rural Tunisia, a special herb tea called "verveine" is made from caraway, fennel creek, and coriander seeds. Special foods such as wheat, barley and/or couscous are eaten in the evening to stimulate the next morning's milk production. In the United States, thistle tea is a known folk remedy used to enhance milk production. It may be problematic, as it contains comfrey. Lac Tea is another product available in health food stores in the United States, which contains nettle, caraway, fennel, and anise and is advertised as an old world recipe to enhance lactation. Guatemalan Indian women take steam baths in the belief that the heat applied to the back increases milk production; they also drink ixbut tea, made from the leaves of euphorbia lancifolia. In addition, hot chocolate is suggested for the first week after the baby is born.

In the south of China, a concentrated soup is prepared to improve the milk supply. It is made of pigs' hooves boiled with ginger preserved in vinegar or wine. Other recipes include tailbones cooked with beans or peanuts or fish tails boiled with papaya or coconut or chicken. The soups are reheated and consumed daily. In the north of China, chicken soup (or tech-

Figure 1.4
Galactogogues (Milk-Producing Substances)

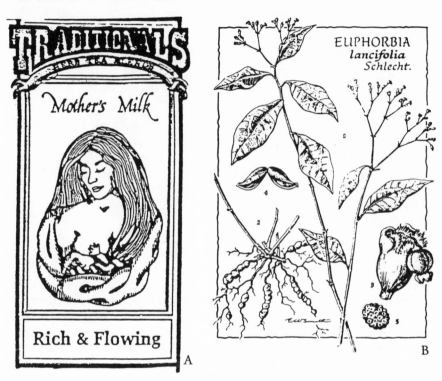

A

B

Mothers in all parts of the world have special foods and drinks they hope will ensure an adequate milk supply. Most of these have not been tested scientifically, but mothers swear by them. Many of the ingredients are similar and are derived from plants, such as: (A) this "milk tea," sold in American health food stores, and (B) the euphorbia plant, which is used as a galactogogue in Guatemala.

nically, adult rooster soup) is commonly used to promote lactation. This special "lactation soup" is consumed for anywhere between two weeks to two months after delivery. Fathers in urban areas have to buy as many as five or six roosters from the rural farmers to be able to make enough lactation soup. Some villagers simply eat whole salt-preserved marine fish, bones and all. In some parts of China, a nursing mother is supposed to eat five to ten eggs per day. For city mothers, many baskets of eggs have to be collected from the countryside. In anticipation of this, the family may save up to three hundred eggs during the pregnancy. Traditional herbs, such as the seeds of the wolf berry and shouwu tuber of the fleece flower, are also added. Chicken millet cooked in red sugar is also prescribed. In Nepal soups of juana seed, fennel, dill, caraway, and cumin are prepared. Also used is a special drink called gendrik made from fermented mushrooms, radishes, and dry greens.

Continents apart, mothers have discovered many of the same herbs, teas, soups, and foods for increasing their milk supply. Many of these recipes have stood the test of time, but western medicine has been slow to verify or dismiss the importance of them. On occasion, a new discovery is triumphantly announced; generally, it turns out to be an ancient folklore utilized for centuries by a so-called primitive society. Some of the ones that have been studied have been found to be nutrient rich in elements that are commonly deficient in the region. For instance, the use of cocoa in the early postdelivery days provides the new mother with a source of iron, zinc, and copper (after pregnancy the mother's iron may be low from blood loss). The cocoa, passed through the mother's milk, may also increase the infant's iron. A concoction made from radish greens in Nepal has been shown to be high in calcium, as is the soup some Chinese use made from pig's hooves steeped in vinegar. As American women (who are told to drink a quart of milk a day before and after a birth) know, calcium is important for a variety of reasons. Calcium helps the blood to clot and assists muscles in working properly, and helps the newborn form strong bones and teeth.

BELIEFS ABOUT COLOSTRUM

Long before the infant is born, the breasts start producing secretions. Some women manually express the early secretions in an attempt to see how far along the pregnancy is. (This is not a particularly good indicator, but it does give you something to do during the nine-month wait.) The yellowness of the colostrum varies according to a woman's diet, although color is not reflective of content. If the mother eats a lot of foods containing Vitamin A and/or carotene, such as palm oil, the secretions may be very yellow. Based on its color, the mother may decide if her milk is good enough for the baby.

Colostrum is increasingly recognized as vitally important for infant health. Sadly, many cultures have been intent on keeping colostrum away from newborns. For a long time it was believed that colostrum was harmful. In many developing countries, mothers distrust colostrum because of its yellow color, believing it to be "pus" or "poison." Newborns were routinely given local concoctions to cleanse and purify them, then nursed by surrogate mothers for as many as twenty days. This was practiced by many peasant societies, save a few such as the New Zealand Maoris, who breastfed from day one.

As far back as the second century BC, Indian Ayurvedic medicine recommended honey and clarified butter for the newborn's first four days, during which the birth mother's colostrum was expressed and discarded. In biblical times, colostrum was also withheld while the infant's bowels were purged with honey until mature milk was present in the mother's breasts. Rose water was used as a purge in the middle ages. In Japan, the elixir *jumi gokoto* was given to the newborn for three days. It was made from a variety of roots and herbs. The ingredients were determined by caste—high borns had ten ingredients, whereas infants of the poor only had five.

Some women give fat or butter to the newborn in the first few days. In Guatemala, surrogate nursing mothers fill in until the biological mother's mature milk comes. In Afghanistan, *fela* (colostrum) is not given to the newborns, but a purge of bitter herbs, sweets, and hyssop seeds are provided instead. Strangely, this practice exists in countries thousands of miles apart, for example, among the Indians of Guatemala and Pakistan and the Africans in Sierra Leone and Lesotho.

The Greeks, Romans, and, later, French and English physicians unquestioningly continued this prelacteal supplementation until the eighteenth century. In 1699, a British physician, Dr. Ettmueller, broke ranks with the medical establishment of the day in recommending colostrum instead of the traditional purge. Neonatal mortality in the eighteenth century was very high in England and Wales, probably due in part to the widespread withholding of colostrum. It was another fifty years before William Cadogan, the "Doctor Spock" of Britain, strongly advocated breastfeeding from birth onwards. Changes concerning traditional beliefs about colostrum slowly began to be reflected in practice. In his "Essay on the Nursing and Management of Children from birth to three years," Dr. Cadogan had this to say about colostrum:

The mother's first milk is purgative and cleanses the child of its long hoarded excrement; no child can be deprived of it without manifest injury. (William Cadogan, 1748)

In the eighteenth century, in England and Wales, the infant mortality was high. It started to drop as more and more doctors promoted early breastfeeding with colostrum and in 1800 the change in infant feeding practices, especially the giving of colostrum, is believed to have caused a 16% drop in mortality (Fildes, 1980).

Even though the positive effects of colostrum are generally acknowledged today, the commitment to ensure that babies fill up on nutrient-rich colostrum is wanting. Soon after birth, infants are commonly given sugar water on a rag or, in the United States, specially prepared sugar water bottles distributed by formula companies. Supplementary feeding of glucose water makes life easier for those staffing hospital nurseries. The sugar water helps keep the babies quiet since it is designed to satisfy their tender appetites and early suckling needs (while also getting them accustomed to a rubber nipple). The reasons typically given for using sugar water is that it is needed to keep the baby from becoming dehydrated or developing low blood sugar until the milk comes in. This practice is totally unnecessary as both conditions are extremely rare. A new baby, even in a hot climate, needs no fluids other than breastmilk (breastmilk is 90% water). Sugar water bottles are harmful as they may cause the baby to lose interest in the breast, thereby reducing the intake of colostrum and with it the sucking that triggers the mother's body to keep producing milk. The innocuous looking bottles actually put the baby at medical risk and sabotage the breastfeeding effort.

There is no question that colostrum is beneficial to the infant and that its anti-infective properties are protective. Even present-day puppy–dog food manufacturers are aware of this and insist that their product should not be used until the puppy has first had colostrum.

PREMATURE AND SMALL INFANTS

Babies are considered premature if they are born from a pregnancy lasting less than thirty-eight weeks. Babies born full term (forty weeks) but weighing less than 5½ pounds are considered to be low birth weight. Regular formula is unsuitable for these infants as their stomachs are too small and their kidneys and liver too immature to digest it. Special formula designed for premature or low birth weight babies must be used in the absence of breastmilk. These babies can only handle small volumes of food, hence they require calorie-dense foods with graded amounts of sodium. While scientists scurry in sterile laboratories debating how standard artificial foods need to be modified for these youngsters, many overlook a simple fact: the breastmilk of mothers with premature infants is the perfect food for premature infants and the breastmilk of mothers with low birth weight infants is the perfect food for low birth weight infants.

Breastmilk is a live fluid that changes according to the needs of the infant. The chemical make-up of the milk of mothers with premature babies is different from that of mothers with full-term infants. Specific constituents of the milk, such as the milk fat, are in forms particularly appropriate for each phase of the baby's life. More digestible fats are in greater proportion when the baby's digestive system is still immature; other fats that provide the basis for brain tissue and central nervous system development are at high levels at an early stage when the baby's brain is growing rapidly.

At Baragwanath Hospital in South Africa, mothers stay in the hospital with their premature infants and feed them breastmilk. If the babies are too small to suck, they are fed expressed breastmilk through a cup; smaller infants are fed intragastrically through a stomach tube. In the bush, where there are not many alternatives, traditional birth attendants have developed ways to handle low birth weight and premature infants. In Malawi, a traditional birth attendant reduced infant mortality in her area by placing low birth weight infants in her own improvised incubator, a cardboard box that ironically had previously contained condensed milk, and added a Coke bottle filled with warm water to provide heat and moisture. For the first few days, she fed the infant sugar water on a rag to establish sucking, then added calorically dense vegetable oil. After three days on this regime, the mothers started breastfeeding and no more low birth weight babies died.

The number of mothers in maternity wards and centers sent home one day after an uncomplicated delivery is increasing. In the United States mothers whose infants are too small or too ill are often sent home because the insurance companies won't pay for them to stay with their babies. These mothers have two options: those who want their infants to have breastmilk can pump their breasts, but then they must travel back and forth several times a day to the hospital to deliver expressed milk (which must be kept refrigerated); or they can dry up their breastmilk with drugs or wait for their breasts to dry up while the hospital staff feed their infants formula. The latter option is usually presented as the prudent one, allowing the mothers to get rest and the hospital staff to feed at their convenience. What the child needs at this point is to be held and fed expressed breastmilk, what the mother needs at this point is to touch and nurture her child. None of these needs get satisfied when the mothers are encouraged to go home and rest so that the hospitals can manage the babies' care.

IS THE MILK GOOD ENOUGH?

Mothers naturally worry about the appearance and volume of their milk. Since antiquity, concerns about the quality and quantity of breastmilk have been voiced. Various "milk tests" have been devised in the hope of finding ways to qualify the substance. In South Africa, many African tribal women felt they could tell how far along their pregnancies were based on the color of milk expressed from their breasts. This "technique" appears to have been used by European women as well (Figure 1.5). In the second century AD, Soranus, a Roman physician, described a "nail test" for milk whereby a drop of milk was placed on the finger nail to judge the milk's quality and consistency. The renowned physician, Paulus Aeginata, added rennet to milk, allowed the cheesy material to settle, and compared the supernatant fluid with the sediment. He was, in fact, precipitating the protein. His analysis was as follows:

Figure 1.5
Gauging the Duration of Pregnancy

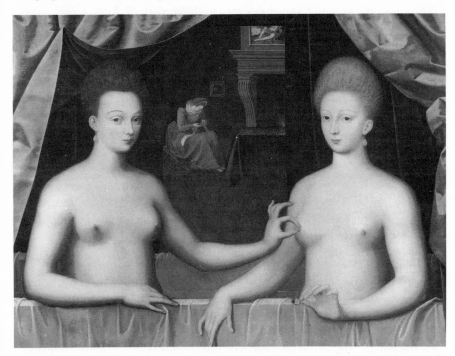

Women in many cultures believe they can gauge the duration of pregnancy by examining the color of their expressed breastmilk. *Photo credit*: Ecole de Fountainebleau, *Gabrielle d'Estrées et sa soeur* (Paris: Musee du Louvre RF 1937-1).

They [the lighter liquid and the sediment] should be roughly equal in quantity; if the latter exceeds the former, the milk will be indigestible; if the opposite occurs, the milk is too weak.

Along with the analysis came the remedies:

If the milk was too thick, the mother should be given emetics to evacuate the phlegm, and if it was offensive, the breastmilk should be expressed and the mother fed on fragrant food and wines.

In Samoa, there is an official milk tester, usually an elderly woman, who puts samples of milk in a dish and adds water and two hot stones. If curdling occurs the milk is pronounced poisoned and suckling delayed. Later the test is repeated, usually with a favorable outcome. A recognized Chinese method for determining the quality of milk is by placing a sample on a special scale used for weighing gold: one pan when full should weigh two "chien" and eight "li."

Thomas Phayer, an English doctor, in *Regiment of Life,* 1546, urged that the milk be examined:

It is good to loke upon the milk and see whether it be thicke and grosse or to much thinne and watrye, blackyshe or bluse or chynge to redness or yellowe for all such is unnatural and evyll. Likewise why ye taste it in your mouth, it be ethyr bytter, salte or sour ye may well peceye it is unwholesome. The milk that is good is whyte and sweate when you drop it on your nail and do move your finger neyther fleteth abrod at every stering wyll hanger faste upon your nale, when you turn downwards, but that which is between both is best.

Numerous beliefs have been promulgated on the nature of breastmilk. For a long time it was believed that breastmilk was actually blood, white in color. The prescription for women who were not producing enough was simple—bloodletting.

Fears of "bad milk" prey on women, at times affecting their milk secretions. In the West, the modern doctor looks neither at the milk nor the mother but focuses instead on the infant's weight. If the infant fails to gain sufficient weight, by the standard charts compiled and distributed by the infant formula companies, it is too often assumed that the mother's milk is inadequate and instructions are given to add formula as a supplement. This thinking is too limited in scope. Even Soranus, eighteen centuries ago, realized that while there could be a problem with the mother's milk (though this is rare), there could also be problems with the mother's health, her psyche, or the baby. The solution is not to blame breastmilk and begin blindly supplementing the infant's diet but rather to search for and address the cause of insufficient weight gain. An inadequate maternal diet, incorrect positioning, and scheduled feeding are some of the factors that need to be considered.

In the early twentieth century, Truby King, a New Zealand physician/ farmer concerned with infant mortality, started training nurses to visit homes and encourage breastfeeding in a "scientific manner." It was Truby King who promoted the harmful practice of nursing babies on a schedule (every four hours) and encouraged mothers to abandon the practice of demand feeding. When mothers were having problems nursing or the infant's weight gain was less than expected, some breastmilk was collected by the nurse and analyzed for fat content. If the mother's milk contained less than 3% fat, supplementary feeding was prescribed. Today, a crematocrit machine (used in the dairy industry) can be used to spin down breastmilk and determine the amount of fat. One American woman, when told by her pediatrician (who did not even examine her breasts or milk) that her milk was no good, changed doctors. Her new physician sent a sample of her milk to a dairy for fat analysis. The note came back, "Dear Mrs._____, If you were one of my herd I would keep you!"

FEEDING STYLES

While it is clear that breastmilk should be offered, how it is offered is a matter of personal choice. There is no standard or ideal position for breast-feeding. Many women sit upright with the baby cradled in their arms, others nurse lying down, while others don't miss a beat, feeding as they walk. The culture and the mother's preference determine feeding positions. Of course, positioning may have to be modified if the mother has had a surgical procedure such as a cesarean section or episiotomy. The latter (cutting the perineum to make the vaginal orifice bigger) is routinely performed in U.S. hospitals; cesarean sections are performed in as many as 25% of American hospital deliveries (at least half of which have been questioned as unnecessary interventions).

Breastfeeding positions vary depending on the culture and attitudes (Figure 1.6). Positions and techniques for breastfeeding have changed and evolved over time. In the sixteenth century, infants were nursed on a table while the mother stood. A modified version of this was used by Georgian, Armenian, and Maronite mothers, who nursed their infants in cradles in the leaning position, supporting themselves by a transverse bar that ran above the cradle. They did not lift the baby after the feed. In Asia, Africa, and Latin America, mothers carry their infants on their backs and swing them around for self-service. Some of the Bush women have been reported to actually throw one of their pendulous breasts over their shoulders to feed an infant strapped on their back (talk about convenience!). In Indonesia, some women feed their infants only on the left breast, as they believe that the left breast contains food while the right breast has only water. Japanese women often feed their infants lying down, as do most mothers who sleep with their infants (this provides the baby with warmth, stimulation, the rhythmical beating of the mother's heart—and milk on demand).

Anthropologist Eva Moloantoa, at the University of Witwatersrand, reporting on the Tswana people in Southern Africa, observed that in African culture many families sleep with the newborn sandwiched between the parents. Among the Tswana people, if the father was not very interested in the baby, it lay on the mother's side and the mother slept in the middle; but where the father was devoted to the child, the infant lay between them. Common beds have been found in cultures around the globe and are still maintained in many parts of the world, including Japan and India.

Sleeping together with the baby at night, which had been the norm since the dawn of human life, fell into disrepute throughout the nineteenth century. Well-intentioned health workers promulgated the importance of sep-

Figure 1.6
Feeding Positions Vary Greatly

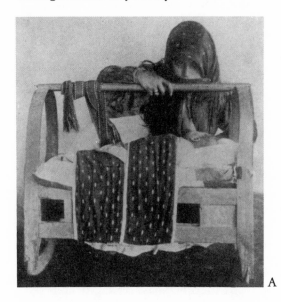

A

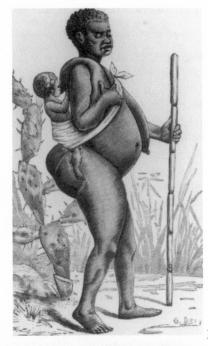

B

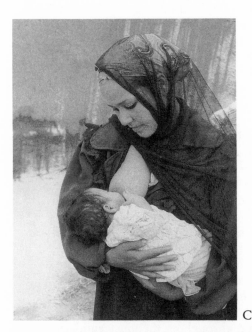

C

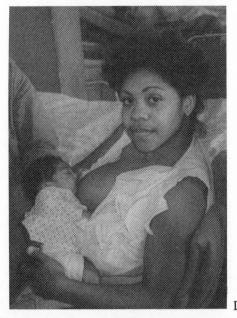

D

Women feed differently (A) Georgian mother standing over a cradle with baby in a fixed position; (B) Bushwoman mother using a self-service approach; (C) Egyptian mother feeding in the Cairo Street; (D) Cuban mother breastfeeding. *Photo courtesy*: (*a*) and (*b*) History of Medicine Division, National Library of Medicine, Bethesda, Maryland; (*c*) UNICEF, Egypt, photo by Ingeborg Lippman; (*d*) Photo by Naomi Baumslag.

arate sleeping and even went as far as passing out banana boxes to serve as cradles. Fears that the baby could be smothered by inattentive parents, or by a breast during a night feeding, were cited as reasons for the separation (there is only questionable evidence of deaths caused by overlaying and there has never been a case reported of a baby being suffocated by a breast). Instead of preventing deaths by suffocation, the health workers actually put the babies at risk for hypothermia. Additionally, infants that are bottle-propped have choked and, in some cases, even suffocated.

Having the whole family sleep together in one bed is and has been quite common in many countries. For centuries in China, the whole family slept in one bed called a *kan*. This was made of bricks which were heated through a stove so the bed was warmed. In urban areas, parents slept with the children until they were seven years of age and attended primary school. In the countryside, the common bed is still used irrespective of age. The normal western sleeping arrangement is based on each individual needing a certain amount of privacy and "space." Expectant parents usually set up the baby's room before the birth. Infants sleep alone in a room separate from their parents often from the first day (where they are separated from their mom and placed in the hospital nursery). Communal-bed babies learn to console themselves with touch and breastmilk; western babies are taught to console themselves with rubber pacifiers and expensive teddy bears (some even with rhythmical ticking "hearts" to simulate the missing mom's heartbeat).

Some families in the United States do maintain a family bed, but it is the exceptional family that values closeness over privacy. The family bed makes breastfeeding much more manageable since no one has to get out of bed and sit up with the child for the nighttime feedings; the mother simply rolls over and, often, goes right back to sleep while the baby suckles.

In addition to not having to extract oneself from the bed and wait for the child to finish feeding (infants consume up to one-third of their daily calories during night feedings), there are also hormonal advantages to feeding the baby on the breast at night. Tine Thevenin explains in *The Family Bed* that the entire time a woman is breastfeeding she is linked chemically to her baby. Breastfeeding mothers notice that they frequently awaken in the middle of the night just before their baby begins to whimper. Results of recent research suggest that a nursing mother may awaken in anticipation of her child's cry because she and her infant dream in unison. It is suspected that the hormone, prolactin, may be the key to this mysterious link. This appears to last only as long as breastfeeding is continued. With bottle-fed infants, this lasts for only about two weeks, after which the mother and child have been chemically separate with different and unequal sleep cycles. The very deep sleep periods are extremely important and essential for restful sleep and a feeling of well-being during waking hours. Since a mother and her nursing infant seem to have equal sleep periods, the mother is able to enjoy some deep, albeit potentially short, sleep periods. The waking of the baby would most likely be during the lighter sleep stages. This may be one of the reasons why nursing mothers do not find nighttime interruptions as objectionable and are not quite as bothered by them as bottle-feeding mothers.

CARRYING BABY

Kangaroo mothers must stare in wonder at us, questioning why they were built with such a superior design. If only human mothers had as intelligent a mechanism as the kangaroos' anatomical pouch that carries their babies safely, keeps them close, is immensely portable, and comes with its own heating system. Adult humans have tried endless techniques for carrying babies. There are front packs, side harnesses, and back carriers. These are designed to keep the hands free, but many adults complain that they cause back pain. The over-the-shoulder sling or wrap, typically used in many traditional cultures, has gained increasing popularity in the United States for infants up to 30 pounds, both because of its simplicity and ease for breastfeeding (as in Figure 1.7). There are also portable baskets to carry, strollers to push, and carts to pull. These, of course, are easier on the back, but they occupy at least one hand, do not provide the baby with the comfort and security of being in physical contact, and are difficult to maneuver on stairs or uneven surfaces. None come close to the convenience of the kangaroo's pouch.

In many traditional cultures, mothers carry their babies on their backs, wrapped in skins, cloths, or shawls. Each mother develops her special way of wrapping her infant. Among the rural Zulu, a head-supporting cuff is sewn on a special cloth carrying blanket, *mbeleko*, to protect the infant's head. Women from South America also carry their babies on their backs in special blankets.

The traditional transportation system for Navaho babies was to be carried around, carefully wrapped, on a cradleboard (called *Awéé Tsaal*). The child's cradleboard was made after the birth because of the fear of making a construction mistake—it was believed that if the back slat was made crooked it would cause the child to be born physically or mentally impaired—so much care was taken in the making of the cradleboard, including an offering of corn pollen and prayers prior to construction. All taboos were carefully observed so as not to cause any harm to come to the infant, considered the most precious of gifts. The back supports and the foot rest were usually made of juniper wood, the head protector fabricated out of oak, and the baby secured to the board with thongs laced to the outer edges of the two back supports. Buckskin thongs were originally used as deer were considered wise, quick, and agile, and it was hoped that the child

Figure 1.7
Carrying Patterns

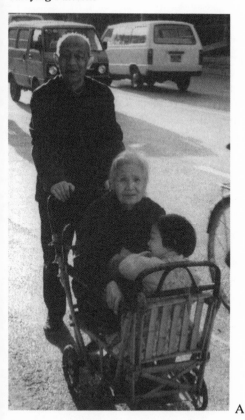

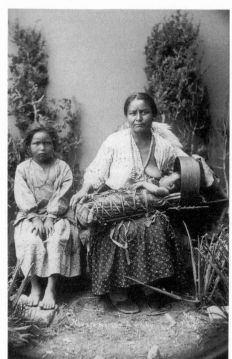

B

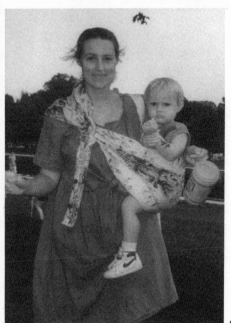

A

C

Devices used to transport children vary from the simple cloth ties to more elaborate structures. (A) This Chinese pushcart was used to transport both infant and grandmother. *Photo courtesy*: Dia L. Michels; (B) Cradleboard used by Navaho mothers. Mothers breastfed while the infant was on the cradleboard. Courtesy Museum of New Mexico, Palace of the Governors, Sante Fe. *Photo courtesy*: Ben Wittick, neg. no. 15724; (C) Modern mother using carrying cloth sling method for transportation. *Photo courtesy*: Naomi Baumslag.

would develop these same attributes. The lacings represented lightning and sun rays; it was believed that warmth would generate from the child because of this. For the Navaho people, the cradleboard was practical and convenient, but it also symbolized the love of a mother for her child.

In some rural areas of Japan, infants were immobilized, with only their heads able to move. In the first few months of life, mothers would hold the wrapped babies against them, providing comfort and warmth (which is important for all babies, especially small ones). As the infants grew, they were carried around in straw baskets.

There is another practical consideration to the use of carriers in developing countries: women often carry heavy loads—in addition to the children. They not only walk for many miles carrying their infants, but water, firewood, and crops as well. Somehow it has been assumed that an infant is almost weightless. One need not carry an infant for long to appreciate that this is a gross miscalculation.

In 1848, Charles Burton, a New Yorker from Greenwich Village whose wife was ill, found carrying his baby around to be too burdensome. To help ease his load, he fashioned a miniature carriage out of a box, four wheels, and a handle. The next day he went out for a stroll pushing his son instead of carrying him. The sight of a father pushing his baby did not go unnoticed. It was too much even for the so-called nonconformists of the day. Newspapers wrote feature stories about it. In a city supporting 20,000 horse-drawn carriages to transport adults, the idea of using a small hand-propelled carriage to transport a child struck everyone as silly, unnecessary, and impractical. People objected that baby carriages would overcrowd sidewalks and be a hazard to pedestrian traffic.

Burton, understanding both the significance of his invention and the tone of public opinion, took his invention to London—where he received the same reaction. That all changed when Queen Victoria heard about it, also understood that it was a good idea, and bought one. Suddenly, perambulators became the height of fashion and Burton became an overnight sensation. He may have returned home weighed down with riches, but he literally lightened the load of millions of parents.

SWADDLING

Since biblical times, and as late as the eighteenth century in Europe, it was fashionable to swaddle babies. Tightly binding a baby's body in cloth or bandages in an attempt to rigidly restrict movement is called swaddling. There have been numerous theories suggested to explain swaddling. Voltaire suspected it was to cut down on the time spent on infant care. Other reasons commonly cited for wrapping infants were to straighten their limbs, to keep them from chills, and to protect them from direct sunlight.

Ruth Benedict, a well-known anthropologist, has speculated that the fundamental values of mothers were, and still are, expressed in their binding techniques. For example, Russian mothers swaddled their infants for two primary reasons: to prevent the weak infant from falling apart and to control the shameful practice of putting toes in the mouth or "handling bad parts." Rumanian women tied the infant's hands to the crib to prevent masturbation. In Greece, infants are swaddled for forty days to help keep the infant's back straight.

Swaddling is not good for children. In addition to hampering normal muscle development and coordination, swaddling can lead to a variety of medical problems involving the lungs, arteries, and veins. Despite growing evidence that swaddling was not a good practice, it has persisted. In the 1740s, William Cadogan, physician to the Foundling Hospital in London, who had radical ideas about giving children breastmilk, sharply criticized the heavy swaddling practices of the day, insisting that infants were not "hot-bed plants" and that "the lighter and looser their clothing the better they would be." One Turkish study found that swaddled infants had a higher incidence of pneumonia. But old habits change slowly. Swaddling is still practiced in limited areas of Eastern Europe, Asia, and the Middle East including Mongolia, Afghanistan, Turkey, and Greece.

DURATION OF BREASTFEEDING

The American Academy of Pediatrics says that babies should be breastfed until age one. . . . It's the lucky baby I feel who continues to nurse until he's two. (Dr. Antonia Novello, U.S. Surgeon General, 1990)

As a global goal for optimal maternal and child health and nutrition, all women should be enabled to practice exclusive breastfeeding and all infants should be fed exclusively on breastmilk from birth to 4-6 months of age. Thereafter, children should continue to be breastfed, while receiving appropriate and adequate complementary foods, for up to two years of age or beyond. (*The Innocenti Declaration on the Protection, Promotion and Support of Breastfeeding*, 1990)

Our nearest relatives, chimpanzees, depend exclusively on breastmilk for about three years and then for another two to three years on a combination of breastmilk and other foods. As late as the 1820s, English women living in East Lincolnshire reportedly suckled their children until they were seven or eight years old. In the Solomon Islands, breastfeeding continued until the children were fifteen. Cultural attitudes, more than any standard for infant nutrition, generally tend to dictate how long women breastfeed.

While there is no question that children should be breastfed, the issue of how long they should be breastfed always provokes lively debate. In every culture, there is an increase in mortality when breastfeeding ceases. This is because the protective properties of breastmilk continue to safeguard the child regardless of age. Once food is introduced, the nutritional and social value of breastfeeding declines. In fact, the value of breastfeeding into or beyond the second year is often neglected, yet the number of pathogens a child is exposed to only goes up as a child becomes older and more active.

Breastmilk is the only food or liquid needed by a child for the first six months. Indeed, the ideal infant diet is exclusive breastfeeding from a healthy woman for a full six months while the immune and digestive systems of the baby continue to mature. Generally, after six months the breastmilk should be supplemented with food to sustain growth. In developing countries, women used to breastfeed for two to three years exclusively, but this has become rare, and even in younger infants exclusive breastfeeding is becoming a rarity. This has become even more rare despite the fact that there are data that in the United States, among well-nourished mothers, infants exclusively breastfed for nine months grow well. In malnourished populations, feeding the mother is key to enabling the infant to breastfeed.

The duration of breastfeeding is largely influenced by cultural pressures. In a bizarre series of events throughout 1991 in Syracuse, NY, a mother had her child taken from her and placed in foster care because it was assumed that her nursing a two year old was somehow tied up with sexual abuse. While all the abuse charges were finally dismissed, a judge found the mother guilty of neglect—for failing to wean her daughter sooner. Only in a culture with no appreciation for breastfeeding could that have taken place. In many parts of the world, a woman would be considered guilty of neglect for weaning a child less than two years old.

In some cultures, the duration of nursing is tied to the gender of the child. Among Iranians, it is traditional to breastfeed girls for two months longer than boys. This is supposed to compensate for the disadvantage a woman has as a result of Moslem religious laws (e.g., daughters inherit half of the property inherited by sons—some compensation . . .). In other cultures, male infants are fed longer than female infants; the male of mixed twins is sometimes given breastmilk while the female is given bottle feeds (often with tragic results) (Figure 1.8). It is a common, but incorrect, assumption that mothers with multiple births cannot produce enough breastmilk. Women with twins and even triplets have successfully fed their babies. In fact, when multiple births do occur, breastfeeding can be lifesaving and a lot less expensive than formula.

Each mother/child team needs to determine for itself how long they are comfortable feeding (sometimes the child refuses to feed before the mother is ready to stop). The only thing that is clear is that there are no rules on the age when the breast should be withdrawn once the child is eating food.

Women all over the world become pregnant and give birth. What is a special, significant experience for each individual woman is a routine fact

Figure 1.8
Girls Are Discriminated against Even in Breastfeeding

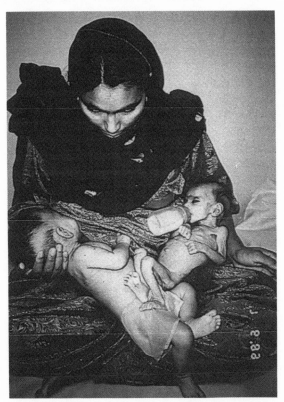

In many societies, the male infant is breastfed longer than the female or given priority. In this case of Pakistani twins, the male was breastfed and the female bottle-fed. The doctor had informed the mother (incorrectly) that she would not have enough milk to nurse both twins. The infant girl died of marasmus. Her brother thrived. "Use my picture, if it will help," said the mother. *Photo courtesy*: UNICEF, Children's Hospital Islamabad, Pakistan.

of life for us as a species. Each baby must be fed and clothed, yet how each child is treated varies widely among, and even within, each culture. Our attitudes toward breastfeeding are indicators of our attitudes toward children. Should children be touched often and encouraged to enjoy the most intimate contact with their mothers, or kept at a distance in an effort to teach them self-sufficiency? Should children be comforted when crying, or be left to exhaust themselves into sleep? Should children be put on a structured schedule, or be allowed to feed and sleep when hungry and tired?

Breastfeeding is not a simple measurable task of inserting calories into a child. Observing how different cultures respond to breastfeeding and knowing the different approaches each culture uses in infant feeding are measures for us to examine methods other than our own. A millennia of human existence has survived because of breastmilk. While no one would wish away the tremendous advances western medicine has offered in maternal and infant health, there is also no need to toss aside all the beneficial knowledge and traditions employed by people in less "modern" cultures. Mothers around the world have long known that *Breast Is Best*, passing that message on from one generation to another with knowledge and practical experiences.

Two

Wet Nursing, Surrogate Feeding, and Healing Qualities of Breastmilk

> Any mother who could afford to hire a wet nurse would never sacrifice her sleep, her social life, her sexual pleasure (intercourse was supposed to interfere with lactation), or her small earnings in the store or shop in order to suckle and care for her own baby. . . . Good mothering is an invention of modernization. In traditional society, mothers viewed the development and happiness of infants younger than two with indifference.
>
> —George D. Sussman, *Selling Mothers' Milk*, 1982

If you mention wet nursing today, most people wrinkle their eyebrows and are not sure what to think, but suspect it is unsanitary at best. The important fact about wet nursing is that before technology and milk surpluses launched the mass production of artificial baby foods, this was the only viable alternative to a birth mother breastfeeding her own child. Dry nursing (as artificial feeding is called) was a death sentence. Wet nursing began as a community's way of saving a baby whose mother could not provide, then "modern" societies turned it into a profession whereby wealthy mothers had the choice not to nurse.

The Pharaohs used wet nurses for rearing their children. Both Moses and Mohammed owed their lives to wet nurses after they were rescued from the bulrushes. In biblical times, the woman who fed the child was considered the real mother even if she was not the biological mother. One example in the Bible is Deborah, who "gave suck" to Rebecca and acted as her surrogate mother. Interestingly, according to the Koran, children suckled by the same nurse are milk sisters and milk brothers; since milk is considered altered blood, they are considered blood relations and are not permitted to marry.

Wet nursing began as a way for one woman to help another woman. In peasant societies, when a mother died, was ill, could not nurse, or had multiple children, close relatives or members of the clan wet nursed her infant(s). It didn't take long, however, for the wet nurse to become a symbol of financial prosperity. Most Egyptians, Babylonians, and Hebrews traditionally breastfed their children for about three years, but the wealthier Greeks and Romans hired slaves to wet nurse. Among the Greeks, special slaves or bondwomen called *duolas* wet nursed for six months and took care of their employer's infants. Cato, the Roman Censor, went even further. He had his wife suckle their servants' children "so they would like him and his better." It did not take long for rich and socially prominent women to employ wet nurses. A fifteenth-century painting by Francoise Clouet, *Diane de Pointier* (allegedly the mistress of Henry the Fourth), shows the subject having a bath while her wet nurse feeds the baby (Figure 2.1). It was in France, in the eighteenth century, that wet nursing reached its peak.

Wet nurses have served as surrogate mothers since the earliest of times. Plato advocated the rearing of all children in crèches by wet nurses, "while taking every precaution that no mother shall know her own child." On the other hand, Roman philosophers and moralists, such as Pliny, Plutarch, and Tacitus, were strongly opposed to wet nursing because they recognized that the attachment between child and wet nurse was so strong that it was often a threat to the natural mother.

One of the most interesting and successful approaches to feeding orphans or discarded infants was in a foundling home in Rome in 1204. Pope Pius III dedicated a large section of the hospital Santa Maria in Sassia (on the banks of the Tiber river) to the care of unwanted infants, infants who hitherto had been thrown into the river. They were left at the home anonymously, and a corps of wet nurses was employed to feed them. Flute and lute musicians played throughout the day to ensure an optimal feeding atmosphere. The infants suckled peacefully, the milk flowed freely (Figure 2.2). When the infants became children, they were trained to play musical instruments and sing and then performed throughout Europe, raising funds for the foundling hospital. Money was also given to young girls who had no dowry, thus enabling them to marry.

In Spain, Italy, and France, high illegitimacy rates led to the establishment of vast foundling hospitals that operated with a revolving container, *tour*, in the door. The baby was placed in the container, ensuring a safe place for the child and anonymity for the parent. Wet nurses served a vital function in foundling homes. They nursed not only their own children but three or four others in addition. In the Paris Maternité Hospital, obstetrician Pierre Budin found that these women nursed as often as thirty-four times a day! It was estimated that the wet nurses produced up to five quarts of milk per day—the greater the demand for their milk, the more they produced. Budin also showed that during an influenza epidemic milk pro-

Figure 2.1
Society Ladies Hired Wet Nurses

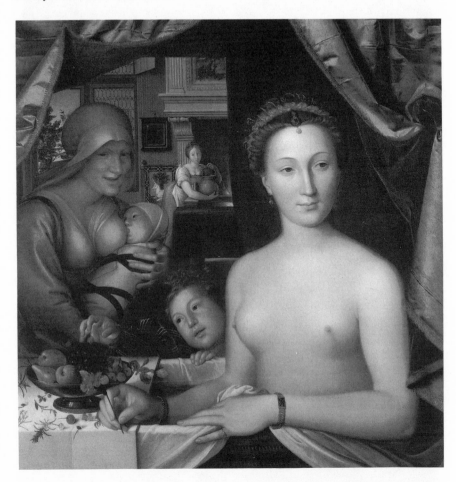

Upper-class women erroneously believed that breastfeeding would permanently alter the shape of their breasts. They failed to realize that pregnancy, not nursing,
altered breast shape. This fifteenth-century painting, by Francoise Clouet, of *Diane
de Pointier* (allegedly Henry IV's mistress) depicts the "virginal" breasts of the
bathing mistress and her wet nurse feeding the swaddled infant. *Photo courtesy*:
National Gallery of Art, Washington, DC, Samuel H. Kress Collection.

duction was decreased (the effect of infection on milk production still has
not been measured).

The early history of wet nursing in France is best documented in the
royal line. All of the French royal children going back at least to the future
St. Louis at the beginning of the thirteenth century were suckled by hired

Figure 2.2
Wet Nurses Breastfed Foundlings to the Tune of the Flute and the Lute

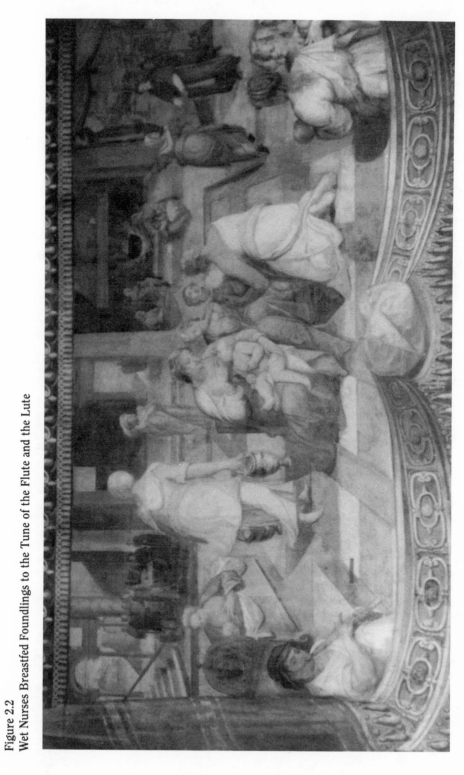

This fresco hangs in the Hospital di Saxii, Rome. *Photo courtesy:* Dr. R.E. Yodaiken.

women, while, in contrast, many foreign princes and princesses were nursed by their mothers. French royal nurses as well as several replacements were kept in reserve after being carefully selected six to eight weeks before the queen was to deliver. The royal babies were nursed for about two years. Their nurses were often changed, either because of lack of milk or as a result of court intrigue. The future Louis XVI had four nurses before he was weaned at the age of twenty-five months. Wet nursing, however, was not restricted to royalty; at social levels below the royal line there was widespread evidence of wet nursing by the twelfth century, which continued into the eighteenth century.

Women in affluent homes hired wet nurses, who were typically women of low social class, some even prostitutes. Wet nursing inherently posed a difficult dilemma: one needed to have recently given birth (it was thought) in order to produce milk, but the wet nurses generally lived with their employer and employees with children were much less sought after. Women seeking these lucrative jobs neglected, abandoned, and even deliberately smothered their own infants so that they could take on the job of breast-feeding someone else's child. In the seventeenth century in France, a law was passed requiring registration of wet nurses, a medical examination (Figure 2.3), and some proof that the wet nurse's own infant was at least nine months old before she could sell her services to someone else. Neglecting an infant became a punishable crime calling for imprisonment of the mother. However, the very law that aimed to keep mother and infant together in its execution often had the opposite effect, since imprisoned women were not permitted to keep their children with them.

In eighteenth-century England, one source of wet nurses was the new lying-in hospitals that were founded through a combination of medical ambition and philanthropy. Only respectable poor women with references could deliver there, and demand for the beds exceeded supply. (Later, some of these hospitals became centers of infection and a feared cause of mother and child death, but when they offered the chance for free food, rest, and assistance in labor, they appealed to the ordinary woman.) More than just providing a service to poor women, they were centers where families could seek wet nurses. The very wealthy made arrangements privately during their pregnancies and would deliberately select a woman who already had a thriving baby as proof of her quality. However, many people had to find a wet nurse in a hurry because a mother had died in childbirth or the original wet nurse had proven unsatisfactory, and they would go to the lying-in hospital where a mother whose baby had died could be hired for wet nursing.

The aristocracy were quick to exploit the fact that the contraceptive effect of breastfeeding could be circumvented by the use of wet nurses, thereby making it possible for their wives to produce a child as often as once a year. Even if a number of the infants didn't survive, as long as the

Figure 2.3
Doctors Examining Wet Nurse Candidates

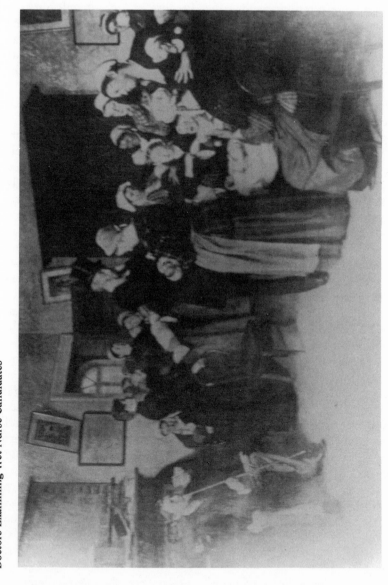

Medical examination of wet nurses became institutionalized in France in the seventeenth century. This painting, *Le Bureau des Nourrices*, by Jose Frappa (1854-1904), from the Musée de l'Assistance Publique in Paris, depicts the medical examination of wet nurses. *Photo courtesy:* Medicine Division, National Library of Medicine, Bethesda, Maryland.

wife did, this strategy gave royal families a chance to acquire large amounts of wealth, power, and influence (by arranging advantageous marriages for the sons and daughters).

Hiring wet nurses did not upset the ladies of high society, as they were anxious to avoid breastfeeding. Many were concerned that breastfeeding would ruin their good health and their figures; they also felt that the constraints of feeding and caring for their children would lead them to neglect their social responsibilities. The society lady was expected to delegate all physical labor to others in order to demonstrate her own superiority and her family's high status. It was as if there were two different species of females: affluent women who were seen as inherently sickly, weak, and especially delicate (not that anyone worried about them going through repeated pregnancies); while working-class women were viewed as the salt of the earth, inherently healthy, strong as horses, and vibrantly robust. Powerful families did not want their women performing the same tedious, daily tasks as ordinary peasant women. Ironically, aristocratic families desired wet nurses for yet another reason—relationships with wet nurses allowed them to cement ties with lower-class women, whose loyalty could be a useful source of information as well as a source of folk medical advice and remedies.

Early America was, of course, settled by people of European background, so it was no surprise that the concept of wet nursing was exported to the New World. Colonial newspapers served as information sources to link employers and employees.

A certain person wants a Wet Nurse to Suckle a child in the House: Inquiries at the Post-Office in Boston. (*Boston News-letter*, July 23–30, 1711)

A wet nurse, who has a good breast of milk only five weeks old, would be willing to suckle a child on reasonable terms. Inquire at the Printers. (*Royal Pennsylvania Gazette*, March 27, 1778)

Wet nursing was not limited to western societies. Around the world, those who could afford wet nurses often did. An example follows of customary arrangements and requirements for hiring a wet nurse in China in 1938:

The employer is expected to pay [the wet-nurse] two months' wages in advance to the wet-nurse when she is engaged, and he agrees to pay a bonus of an extra month's wages after the child is weaned. She is expected to serve a probationary period of three days to a week in the home. After her wet-nursing duties are completed in the one family, she may be taken on as a servant, she may seek further employment as a wet-nurse, or she may return to her own home. It is considered desirable that the wet-nurse should have certain qualities. She should be young, healthy, of pleasant disposition, and if possible of pleasing appearance. A primiparous woman is preferred. Her breast development should be ample, and her attention is paid to the areola of the nipples, which should be black as an indication of the recent delivery of the nurse's own infant. It is recognized that the milk must be white and thick. (Platt and Gin, "Chinese Methods of Infantfeeding and Nursing," 1938)

In today's society, one often hears the lament that the wealthy educated families have only one or two children while the poor people on welfare keep breeding. The situation in the eighteenth century allowed for exactly the reverse. Wealthy women hired poor women to wet nurse their children. While the infants missed out on their biological mothers' milk, these new mothers lost the natural birth control effects associated with lactation. It was the upper-class women who often had large numbers of closely spaced infants, while the poor wet nurses spent much less time with their partners (since they often lived with their employers) and enjoyed an extended period without ovulation from the lactation. This situation allowed the wealthy woman to function as a supplier of heirs, but at a cost—with the repeated pregnancies came a correspondingly high maternal (and infant) mortality.

Wet nursing could be regarded as a terrible example of the exploitation of women—a chilling example of a society that condoned a woman neglecting her own child so she could care for the baby of a rich woman. But wet nursing also provided a status job and financial security in a culture offering very few safe, lucrative jobs to uneducated women. The wet nurse was more family than servant, and the job required no specialized schooling or social connections. In addition, it paid quite well. What's more, if the heir raised by the wet nurse thrived, the family felt obligated to her and generally took care of her through old age. A royal wet nurse who successfully weaned her charge could look forward to being promoted to a permanent position in the court.

Of course, although wet nursing provided many solutions, it also brought its own set of problems. There was concern that a variety of diseases could be transmitted to the children through the nurse. Some wet nurses were promiscuous, expensive, or meddled in family affairs. Some appear to have had difficulty nursing their charges and, to fatten them, fed them malt liquor; to quiet them, drops of opium. Opium was either given to the child by mouth or applied to the woman's nipple. (This type of supplementation was not unique to wet nurses; mothers, too, have been reported to give opium to their infants to ensure a bit of peace.)

All wet nursing was not done in the homes of the employers. It was not uncommon for infants to be sent to wet nurses in the country, hence the terms "baby farm" and "farmed out." Part of the rationalization for this was that infants would do better in the fresh country air. This notion of a peaceful country existence was, to a large degree, wishful thinking—parish records show a high rate of infant mortality in such situations.

Despite these difficulties, fashionable women continued to use wet nurses. Anthony Trollope, a Victorian novelist, expressed the feeling of the day regarding fashionable women in this passage in his novel *Doctor Thorne*, published in 1858:

Of course Lady Arabella could not suckle the young heir herself. Ladies never can. They're gifted with the powers of being mothers. Nature gives them bosoms for show, but not for use. Lady Arabella hired a wet nurse.

High society ladies erroneously believed that nursing would ruin their figures. In fact, breastfeeding women lose the pregnancy weight more easily than women who do not nurse. There are innumerable examples of "ladies of society" (Figure 2.4) who have breastfed, fulfilled their social obligations, and maintained their good shape, such as Princess Grace of Monaco, who nursed all her children.

Many wet nurses were held in high esteem by their grown nurslings. The French physician Jacques Guillemeau, in his book *Nursing of Young Children* (1612), tells of a boy who greeted his nurse with gold, but only gave silver to his mother because she had no alternative but to nourish him in her womb, whereas the nurse carried him three years in her arms and "nourished me with her own bloude."

Another legendary wet nurse was Judith Waterford, who in 1831 celebrated her eighty-first birthday by demonstrating that she could still squeeze milk from her breast, milk which was "nice, sweet and not different from that of young and healthy mothers." In her prime she produced two quarts of breastmilk unfailingly every day, but admitted sorrowfully that after the age of seventy-five she could not have managed to breastfeed effectively more than one infant at a time.

SELECTION OF WET NURSES

Those who hired wet nurses expected candidates to meet certain physical and social criteria, many highly subjective and some irrational. Sixteenth-century European guidance for the selection of an ideal wet nurse was derived mainly from classical Latin sources and required that the ideal candidate:

Should be of healthy lineage, good behaviour, sober, even-tempered, happy, chaste, wise, discreet, careful, observant, understanding, conscientious, and always willing to give the breast. She should be physically healthy with a pleasing countenance "ruddie mouth" a rosy complexion "verie white teeth" and broad but not pendulous breasts with good nipples.

Figure 2.4
Society Lady Breastfeeding

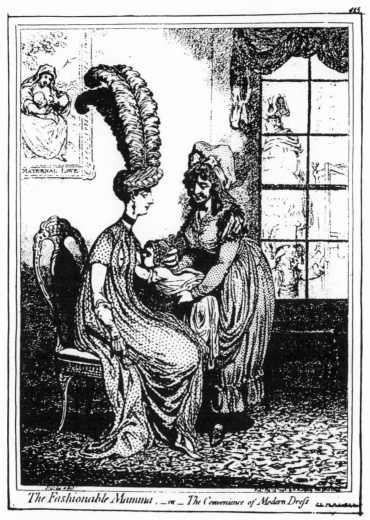

The Fashionable Mamma . — or — The Convenience of Modern Dress

Source: Etching by James Gillray (1756–1815). *Photo courtesy*: Wellcome Centre Medical Photographic Library, M13937.

According to Wickes, the desirable characteristics of a good wet nurse have been slavishly copied from book to book up to 150 years ago. Perhaps they have never been more pleasingly recounted than by S. de Saint-Marthe, who wrote the *Paedotrophia* in Latin in 1584, which was translated into English by W. H. Tyler in 1797.

Chuse one of middle age, nor old or young and strong.
Nor plump nor slim her make, but firm and strong.
Upon her cheek, let health refulgent glow
In vivid colours, that good humor shew:
Long be her arms, and broad her ample chest:
Her neck be finely turn'd, and full her breast:
Let the twin hills be white as mountains of snow.
Their swelling veins with circling juice flow:
Each in a well projecting nipple end.
And milk, in copius streams, from these descend:
This the delighted babe will instant chuse.
And he best knows what quantity to use.
Remember too, the whitest milk you meet.
Of grateful flavour, pleasing taste and sweet,
Is always best; and if it strongly scent
The air, some latent ill the vessels vent
Avoid what, on your nail too ropy proves.
Adheres too fast, or thence too swiftly moves.

Wet nurses were expected to eat and live "right"—warned against bad air, bad smells, salty spiced foods, garlic, mustard, stale cheese and also roast meat if the infant's complexion is moist and phylegmatic. . . . Told to "spurn all raw fruit and drink only ale, beer, barley, water or wine, rest whenever, . . . keep bowels open and shun all disquietness of mind." (Wickes, 1953)

At one point, the color of the wet nurse's hair was used as a criterion of fitness to nurse. One preposterous research study attempted to show that the composition of breastmilk of women with brown hair was of a higher quality than the milk produced by women with red or blonde hair (Table 2.1). Yet another notion was that blondes had sanguine temperaments and as a consequence the milk of blondes was apt to become altered under mental excitement. There was no basis for these contentions, and no one knows how many perfectly good women were deprived of a lucrative job on the basis of these "research" findings. Later, smoking was added to the list of forbidden activities—this was one of the few reasonable measures advocated. The size of the breast, incidentally, is of no consequence; all breasts have the necessary glands—the ability to produce milk is independent of breast size.

It was correctly felt that the milk was a channel for more than just nutrition. Medical examinations were often required and were useful in helping to rule out unhealthy women, those with alcohol and drug addictions, and those deemed mentally unstable. (It was assumed that tuberculosis and syphilis could be transmitted to the infant through the wet nurse. They can, but the milk is not the vessel of transmission. Tuberculosis is transmitted

Table 2.1
Analysis of a Blonde and a Brunette Wet Nurse's Milk (both aged 22)

	Blonde		Brunette	
Constituents	Sample 1	Sample 2	Sample 1	Sample 2
Water	892.0	881.5	853.3	853.0
Solids				
butter	35.5	40.5	54.8	56.0
casein	10.0	9.5	16.2	17.0
milk sugar	58.5	64.0	71.2	70.0
salts	4.0	4.5	4.5	4.0

Data were used to illustrate that blondes were not good milk producers; data were extrapolated to redheads, who were considered the most unsuitable wet nurses. Much misinformation was spread from this "scientific study."

Source: J.F. Simon, "Mother's Milk and its Chemical and Physiological Properties," Ph.D. diss., Berlin, 1838.

through droplet infection; syphilis can be transmitted through infected sores.)

At one stage, it was believed that personality traits and temperament could also be passed through the milk. This led to some interesting situations. On American plantations in the South, before the Civil War, it was common for black "nannies" to feed white infants as well as their own. Nevertheless, the racial prejudice of some whites was strong enough to preclude the use of black nannies as wet nurses for fear that the white children would grow up speaking with the accents of black slaves and using their mannerisms.

Commercial wet nursing became less popular for a variety of reasons. Fear of transmission of syphilis through the milk, although suspected as early as the fifteenth century, increased significantly in the seventeenth century. By the end of the nineteenth century, wet nursing had fallen into disrepute. Moralists, child advocates, and improvements in public health all helped spur the move from "wet" to "dry" nursing. Dry nursing had been lethal. For example, in 1829, the Dublin Foundling Hospital was closed down because 99.6% of the babies died; all the infants had been artificially fed.

As chlorinated water, better sewage disposal, as well as the introduction of sterilizable bottles, rubber teats, and so-called milk substitutes became available in the late nineteenth and early twentieth centuries, infant-feeding attitudes started changing. Some moralists claimed that a bottle would be less of a rival for the child's affections and (the bottle's) moral qualifications compared to those of a wet nurse were simply sublime. Doctors began postulating about the problems of breastmilk. One doctor, referring to the mechanism of the mammary gland, felt "when this mechanism is interfered with, good milk may also become a poison to the infant. . . . [It] is evident therefore that there is nothing ideal about breastmilk." Artificial feeding made possible the replacement of the wet nurse with the newly revered "pocket nurse"—a nanny with a glass bottle and a rubber teat.

SLAVES AS BREEDERS AND FEEDERS

In some parts of eighteenth-century American society, a household was not complete without a cadre of slaves. The duties of some of the female slaves included breeding and breastfeeding.

Wet nursing is usually associated with the aristocracy. Ironically, some slaves had wet nurses. Pregnant female slaves were seen as an economic resource—each slave produced at home was one more you didn't have to buy at the market. Baby slaves had the added attraction that you could raise them as slaves and not have to beat them into docility as adults. The black women who were considered good breeders were given baby slave production as part of their duties. These women were, in turn, provided wet nurses (often elderly slaves) to increase both their infant survival rate and their fertility. So commonly were female slaves used as breeders, that rules for the protection of these women and their children were explicit:

Sucklers are not required to leave their children at the children's house before going to the field. The period of suckling is twelve months. Their work lies always within half a mile of their quarters. They are required to cool before commencing to suckle—to wait 15 minutes at least in the summer, after reaching the children's house before nursing. They are allowed 45 minutes at each nursing to be with their children. They return three times a day until their children are 8 months old—in the middle of the morning, at noon and in the middle of the afternoon. The amount of work done by the suckler is about 3/5 of that done by a full hand, a little increased toward the last. . . . Pregnant women at 5 months are put on the sucklers gang. No ploughing or lifting must be required of them. (Blanton, 1931)

The slaves were doing more than feeding their own children. While "fruitful Virginia wives" produced baby after baby (only a high mortality rate kept the households within bounds), it was black wet nurses who fed and cared for the young white children. The white mothers' lack of breastfeeding was undoubtedly partly responsible for the high birth rates. The black wet nurse played an important role in these large families.

DO YOU HAVE TO HAVE A BABY TO BREASTFEED?

It is commonly believed that lactation only occurs following conception and birth, but this is not necessarily so. Certain species such as elephants and foxes lactate and suckle young without ever giving birth. For humans, continued suckling over a period of time is the requirement to stimulate milk production—pregnancy is not necessary.

Many women who have breastfed can begin again by simply initiating sucking. Women who have never given birth but who wish to breastfeed can also do so. In many cases, women who have adopted infants and young children have successfully breastfed them. When an arrival date is known, lactation consultants suggest women pump their breasts several times every day for two-to-three months before the baby arrives. In many cases, no milk is seen during the entire pumping period, but it begins to flow as soon as the baby latches on.

Another technique is to "breastfeed" the child formula, using one of the devices on the market for this purpose, such as a Lact-Aid. The mother puts formula in a pouch that is connected to a thin tube, and secures the pouch above the breast, typically on one shoulder (it looks similar to a hospital intravenous feeding set-up). The tube is then attached to the nipple; as the child sucks on the nipple, the mother's breast is stimulated, the baby receives a feeding, there is no issue of nipple confusion, and the two share the skin-to-skin contact and closeness of nursing. As the mother's milk comes in, the feeding device is eliminated.

SURROGATE FEEDING

Two other methods of wet nursing, still practiced today and often informally, are cross nursing and surrogate feeding. Cross nursing occurs when mothers breastfeed each other's children; for example, while one mother works, the other feeds (and vice versa); when baby-sitting; or in times of crisis. In cultures that are very family oriented, surrogate feeding may take place and generally involves one of the grandmothers caring for, and even breastfeeding, the children so that the parents can maintain full participation in the work force. Such was the case in the Bible when Naomi served as wet nurse to the infant of her daughter-in-law, Ruth. This practice of grandmothers breastfeeding is not uncommon in many parts of Africa. Grandmothers may take herbs orally and even apply them to the nipples in order to accelerate the onset of lactation.

We now understand how breastmilk production works, but, historically, western-trained researchers have had great difficulty accepting such "abnormal lactation." Margaret Mead's findings support this:

In 1933, when I returned from New Guinea and reported that women, some of whom had never borne children and others who had not lactated for many years could suckle newborn children, I was challenged with the query: How do you know they produced milk? I could only reply that it was a substance, white in colour, emitted by the maternal breast, on which the infant lived and thrived. My evidence consisted of two pairs of identical twins; in each case, one twin was fed by its own mother and the other twin was fed by an adoptive mother in whom lactation had been induced by the combination of the infant's suckling, forced fluids, and a definite intention.

Several articles in the medical literature have reported on this phenomenon. A piece in the *Dictionaire de Sciences Medicale* told of a woman sixty-eight years old, who offered her breast to an infant whose mother had recently died, and soon had sufficient secretions of milk to support the child. A story in an 1874 *Charleston Medical Journal and Review* tells of a woman sixty years of age who offered her breast, in play, to an infant, and was surprised after three weeks of this amusement to find that she began to secrete milk in excess of its young mother.

Though it may seem strange that a grandmother, or even a woman who has never been pregnant, can produce milk, it is more surprising that there are a few reported cases in the literature of men suckling their infants and even producing breastmilk. There are a handful of stories relating this particular type of "abnormal lactation." One story, told in *Voyages to the Polar Sea*, involved a Chippewa Indian who, on losing his wife in childbirth, put the infant to his own breast, earnestly praying that he might be able to nourish it and eventually producing enough milk to do so. Another story is of the thirty-two-year-old South American peasant whose wife died in childbirth and who reportedly sustained the child with his own milk. A story in the *British Medical Journal*, published in 1884, reported how a highly emotional man disturbed by his wife's suffering in childbirth fell ill, experienced fullness and pain in his breasts, and began to secrete milk. Male patients with liver disease have been known to secrete a milk-like fluid from their breasts. Clearly, the physiological activities of the mammary glands and the mechanisms by which they are controlled are complex.

BREASTMILK PUMPS

Milk can be expressed very effectively by hand by simply squeezing the breasts correctly, but efforts to find mechanical devices for extracting the milk have been underway for hundreds of years. Women pump out their breastmilk to create a supply of food for the infant that can be used when the mother is not willing or able to nurse (Figure 2.5). While pumping can be time consuming, most women find it is a relatively simple process.

Today, there are a large number and variety of breast pumps on the market, falling into three categories: manually operated pumps, battery and small electric pumps, and heavy duty electric pumps. All the pumps induce the milk to come out by using a rhythmic suction action. Manual pumps are the most portable and least expensive option; heavy duty electric pumps are highly effective and can pump both breasts simultaneously—they are particularly good for maintaining a milk supply over a long period of time. These pumps are heavy and expensive; they are typically found in nursing centers and can be rented for home use. Increasingly, employers are providing pumping stations for their employees. The Clinton White House has recently established such a station, setting a new milestone for facilities available to White House staff. In another trend-setting move, Amoco Corporation announced that it is now supplying lightweight miniaturized breast pumps to nursing employees who must travel.

Human breast pumps have provided flexibility for countless numbers of women. They have also been used as veterinary aids to help animals born in captivity into a successful nursing relationship. One such incident occurred when Pearl, a 6,500-pound Asian elephant in the St. Louis Zoo, gave birth to Raja, a healthy male calf. Pearl was unfamiliar with breastfeeding. Her breasts became engorged and her baby hungry. Using a double-breast heavy duty electric pump, zoo staff, with the help of Diana Estep, a local lactation consultant, pumped Pearl's breasts every three hours, enabling baby Raja to consume over thirty-seven cups of milk a day. Once Pearl relaxed into the pumping routine and Raja relaxed into a feeding routine, the zoo staff were able to successfully encourage Raja to latch on, establishing a nursing relationship that would last for the next three to four years.

BREASTMILK BANKS

Expressed breastmilk can be fed to the mother's child, but it can also be made available for other infants. Feeding infants donated breastmilk, which is called cross or surrogate feeding, is another alternative to wet nursing. Pumped milk, either fresh or frozen, is used to feed infants who have lost their mothers or whose mothers cannot breastfeed. Breastmilk banks, which pool milk from a number of donors, provide an invaluable service to infants who would not otherwise experience the benefits of breastmilk. Breastmilk banks are the vehicle that typically matches up milk from donors with infants who need it. Most commonly located in hospitals, breastmilk banks are also available in daycare centers in some parts of the world.

Figure 2.5
Breast Pumps

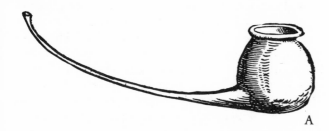

A

Rubber Teething Rings.

No. 8R612

No. 8R609 Rubber Teething Rings, seamless, full size, best white rubber. Price, each.........3c
No. 8R613 Rubber Teething Rings, full size, seamless best black rubber. Price, each...3c
No. 8R615 Bone Teething Ring, 1¾ inches, nicely finished. Price, each..........4c

No. 8R618 Vegetable Ivory Teething Ring. Teething ring of real vegetable ivory and large seamless black rubber nipple
Price, each.........10c

No. 8R621 New Style Rubber Teething Ring, with one hard and one soft nipple, a great favorite with babies.
Price, each......... 20c

If by mail, postage extra, each, 2 cents.

Nursery Bottle Fittings.

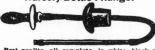

Best quality, all complete, in white, black or maroon.
No. 8R624 Price, each............................5c

Nursing Flasks.

Graduated to hold 8 ounces, oval shape with sloping sides. No corners, therefore easy to clean.
No. 8R627 Price, each..........6c
Weight, 14 oz.

Plain Nursing Bottle.

No. 8R630 Plain Nursing Bottle, for tube fittings. Each 5c
If by mail postage extra, each, 14 cents.

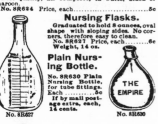

No. 8R627

THE EMPIRE

No. 8R630

Nursing Bottles.

Nursing Bottles. Burr patent white rubber fittings.
No. 8R648 Price, each..........8c
If by mail, postage extra, each, 15 cents.

S., R. & Co.'s Complete Nurser.

S., R. & Co. Nurser No. 1. Fitted with white, black or maroon fittings. Complete with two brushes in each box. Weight, 16 oz.
No. 8R651 Price, each..........17c

S R & CO.

Rubber Nipples.

Rubber Nipples for tube fittings. White, black and maroon.
No. 8R633 Price, per dozen, 20c; each......2c
Rubber Nipples to fit over bottle. White, black or maroon.
No. 8R636 Price, per dozen, 25c; each......3c

Rubber Nipples, Davidson's patent. Black, white or maroon. To fit over bottle.
No. 8R639 Price, per dozen, 30c; each.... 3c

Health Nipples. Made from the finest Para rubber; is constructed so that the infant can obtain a strong hold and renders nursing easy.
No. 8R642 Price, per dozen, 45c; each......4c

PAT'D. APL-10-88.

Mispah Valve Nipple. Making nursing easy. Allows the food to flow easily. Prevents colic.
No. 8R645 Price, per dozen, 50c; each......5c

If by mail, postage extra, per dozen, 6 cents; each, 1 cent.

Glass Nipple Shields.

Glass Nipple Shield with white rubber nipple and bone guard.
No. 8R654 Price, each....8c
If by mail, postage extra, each, 8 cents.

Glass Nipple Shield with long flexible rubber tube, mouth guard and rubber nipple.
No. 8R657 Price, each..........10c
Weight, 8 ounces.

English Breast Pump.

English Breast Pump, with white rubber bulb. One in box.
No. 8R660 Price, each...16c
If by mail, postage extra, each, 8 cents.

B

(A) A sixteenth-century breast pump, probably one of the first to be devised. *Photo courtesy*: History of Medicine Division, National Library of Medicine, from W.H. Ryff, *Frawen-Rosengarten* (Frankfurt: C. Engenolff, 1548); (B) Advertisements in the 1902 Sears catalogue show the bottles, nipples, and breast pumps available at the beginning of this century. *Photo courtesy: Sears, Roebuck Catalogue,* 1902 edition (Avenel, NJ: Gramercy Books, 1993).

Many breastmilk advocates argue that there is no need for formula to exist. Mothers should feed their own children, either in person or with a supply of pumped milk, and in the few instances where this is not possible, the child should be fed donated milk obtained from breastmilk banks.

Both Sweden and Denmark have active bank programs. "Milk kitchens" located in the dietary departments of hospitals store containers of tested and pooled breastmilk for nursery use. Swedish milk banks accept breastmilk expressed within the first three months of lactation and pay the equivalent of about $21 per liter, tax free. Donors provide an average of 50 liters each. Danish milk banks accept milk expressed through the fourth month and also pay donors by the liter.

The Eastern European countries, so often associated with crude medical services before the end of the Cold War, have operated some of the most successful breastmilk banks in the world. The combination of disdain for formula and a lack of sufficient hard currency to rely on imported artificial foods resulted in significant efforts being funneled into the creation and support of elaborate networks and policies to supply and use pooled breastmilk. Since the end of World War II, women have been donating breastmilk for use in hospital-run milk banks. In 1989, over 200,000 liters of mother's milk were collected in the eastern part of Germany. In the (formerly East) German town of Leipzig, ninety-three women supplied 10,000 liters of milk a year, each donating between a pint and a quart a day. The women were given a small amount of compensation, medical tests prior to becoming donors, and they, along with their partners, were instructed in ways to minimize infections and how to practice low-risk behaviors. The milk was routinely tested microbiologically and screened for alcohol and nicotine.

Pooled expressed milk was given to small, sick, and premature infants who were not receiving enough milk from their biological mothers. Any infant under nine months old, admitted with any disease whatsoever, and all postsurgical pediatric patients were given banked milk to reduce the risk of inflammation and infection. Mothers of children with cow's milk allergy were also given daily supplies of pooled bank milk for home use. In these rudimentary hospital environments—where nothing is disposable, equipment is minimal, and cleanliness is shoddy—the children fed on human breastmilk had significantly lower infection rates than in the most technologically sophisticated western hospitals.

In the United States there are eight human milk banks and there is one in Canada that store and supply donated pooled human milk. The milk is required for infants who are premature, allergic to cow's milk, have intractable diarrhea, and those with immune deficiencies. All the donors are screened for HIV and hepatitis. Donor milk is now pasteurized as a preventive measure against the spread of AIDS. Unfortunately, this process destroys much of the protective anti-infective properties of milk.

Many hospitals still rely on breastmilk banks for some of their infant food needs; unfortunately, fear of spreading AIDS through the breastmilk and lack of funding have forced many of the world's milk banks to shut down. The few remaining have begun pasteurizing the milk. One such milk bank in Finland found infection rates in infants rose within a short time of implementing pasteurization. Similarly, Canadian hospitals experienced several major outbreaks of infection and several avoidable infant deaths within months of closing down their milk banks.

Despite all the restrictions on the use of breastmilk, there now appears to be a renewed interest in milk banks, especially for premature infants. In some institutions, the milk is "fortified," depending on the prevailing medical fashion. The milk is also used for infants who are allergic to cow's milk. Of note is the fact that, to date, there have been no cases of AIDS reported from the use of pooled milk from milk banks.

INTERSPECIES NURSING

Babies have enjoyed their mother's milk from time immemorial, but the notion of drinking the milk of another animal took some time to take hold. The Greeks and Romans commonly referred to the barbarians as "milk drinkers" (the Greek word was *galaktopotes*), so remarkable did this habit seem to them. In the fifth century BC, the Greek historian Herodotus described the Massagetai, inhabitants of the Caucasus, in this way: "They sow no crops but live on livestock and fish, which they get in abundance from the river Araxes; moreover, they are drinkers of milk!"

Eventually, the idea of sharing milk among species did take hold. In the quest to provide infants with breastmilk, it was attempted to feed infants directly from the teats of animals (most people are familiar with this concept from Rudyard Kipling's *The Jungle Book*, in which a baby boy, named Mowgli, is abandoned in the jungle and successfully raised on wolf's milk). In the seventeenth century, sick infants and foundlings were fed on asses' and goats' milk (Figure 2.6). Alphonse Le Roy, in 1775, instituted a policy in his hospital for foundlings to suckle directly from goats. He explained:

Each goat [who] comes to feed enters bleating and goes to hunt the infant which has been given to it, pushes back the covering with its horns and straddles the crib to give suck to the infant. There is in milk besides different nutritious principles an invisible element, the element of life itself, a fugitive gas which is so volatile that it escapes as soon as the milk is in contact with the air. This is why it is impossible to rear infants with animal milk or milk which has been expressed from the breast.

Asses were also used as wet nurses and some infants were fed directly with asses' milk. At the Hospice des Enfants Malades, the animal stalls were

Figure 2.6
Infants Feeding Directly Off Domestic Animals

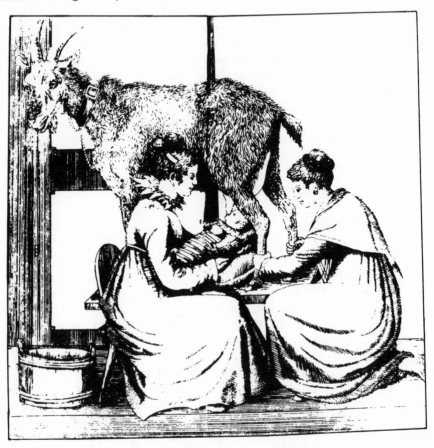

In the seventeenth century, it was fashionable for sick infants and foundlings to be fed animal milk. The animals were even kept in stables adjacent to the hospital ward, and infants were often fed directly off the animals. The outcome was usually fatal. *Source*: G.J. Witkowski, *Histoire des Accouchements chez Tous les Peuples* (Paris: Steinheil, 1887). *Photo courtesy*: History of Medicine Division, National Library of Medicine, Bethesda, Maryland.

directly across from the wards; elaborate procedures were developed to maintain regular interspecies feeding.

Goats as wet nurses have been used worldwide. The Bedouins still resort to the use of a goat or sheep when no human nurse is available. The Hottentots in Southern Africa tied their nurslings under goats' bellies so they could feed there. Goat's milk was chosen as a human breastmilk substitute because goats were easier to obtain and cheaper than human wet nurses. Pigs have also been used as wet nurses, but less so. In parts of Peru, two types of milk drinks for children were made, one from a black burro (used for a soothing tonic) and another from a dog (to build a good and strong stomach). Around the turn of the eighteenth century, limited chemical analysis of milk was possible; from this it was determined that asses' milk was closest in composition to human milk. Goat's milk came in second. Cow's milk came into popular usage only because it was inexpensive and easy to come by, not because it was particularly high in quality or particularly appropriate for infants.

This tradition of infants feeding from animals stems from biblical times, when infants were fed from the teats of camels. The story of Romulus and Remus, who were given wolf's milk, is an oft-quoted success story, but in reality many infants fed directly from animals did not survive. Using animals as wet nurses was not only difficult logistically, but the results of this form of artificial feeding were often disastrous.

Not only have animals been used to feed humans, but humans have, and still do, feed animals (Figure 2.7). Animals have been nursed by women for a variety of reasons, including to aid destitute animals, to relieve engorged breasts, to prevent conception, to promote lactation, and to develop "good nipples"—to name a few. Ancient Romans and Persians put animals to the breast; the custom is still reported among Neapolitans and roving gypsies of Transylvania, Germany, New Zealand, Australia, Sumatra, Thailand, Japan, and South America. Travelers have observed women in British Guiana nursing not only their children of different ages, but also their four-footed brethren, just as obligingly and with equal tenderness. In parts of Africa, such as the Cameroons, in New Guinea, and among Amazon Indians, some women suckle domestic puppies and piglets. This evidently was also practiced in Canada, where Indian women often suckled young dogs and Puma Indians and reportedly withdrew their breasts sooner from their own infants than from their puppies.

In Persia and Turkey, young dogs were put to the breasts to toughen the nipples and to make them better for the infant to suck. Wet nurses in Turkey used suckling puppies to maintain their milk supply if they had to travel by sea from distant villages to the capital. In Dauphine, France, where children were nursed 2½–3 years to help prevent another pregnancy, if the child died too soon, another child or a puppy was used as a replacement. It has even been reported (by Friedrich Osiander, in 1799) that young dogs were suckled by women in Gollinger to disperse obstinate breast nodules. In America, Davies (the first American pediatrician) recommended regular application of a strong puppy, from the seventh month of pregnancy, to harden and conform the nipples, improve breast secretion, and prevent inflammation. He advised, "The puppy's suckling efforts if started early enough prepared the nipples for future assaults of the child." For

Figure 2.7
Women Breastfeed Animals

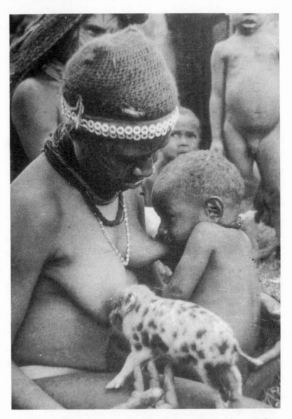

In New Guinea, a mother breastfeeds her infant
alongside the piglet she is fattening for a feast. This
is socially acceptable in this culture. *Photo courtesy*:
Dr. C.D. Williams.

women too modest to make use of a puppy and so unfortunately organized
as to lack nipples altogether or have them short or sunken in, he recommended drawing them out daily with a large tobacco pipe.

In an efficient household, feeding both the animals and babies could be
done simultaneously. This has also been reported in bottle-fed infants.

Stories of interspecies nursing are not limited to Disney fables, foreign
lands, or centuries past. In *Wild Brother: Strangest of True Stories from
the North Woods* (Little, Brown, 1921), William Lyman Underwood tells
of a Vermont family that took in a bear cub whose mother was killed near
a logging camp. The family cherished the bear as a family member until
his behavior became too dangerous and unpredictable. They then sent him
to a zoo.

These stories underscore the importance of breastfeeding for survival—for all mammal species.

NURSING THE AGED

Breastfeeding is usually associated with women nourishing infants. But in addition to nursing their own children, acting as surrogate nurses, and nursing animals, women have also been known to nurse the sick, the aged, and the imprisoned (Figure 2.8). This appears to be particularly so in cultures where the aged are revered. Evidence of this is found in Chinese, Japanese, and even in some American literature. One Chinese story indicates that on her death bed, an old lady blessed her dutiful daughter-in-law who had kept her alive for several years with her daily dose of breastmilk as a "health food." Thomas Moffet, in 1655, penned the following advice in *Health Improvement*: "Neither is a woman's milk only for young and tender infants but also for men and women in ripen years fallen by age or sickness into such positions and suggest asses milk as alternative."

The literature has many examples of breastmilk use in the aged. In Steinbeck's *Grapes of Wrath*, when the family reached California, completely destitute, they were visited by an old, sick, starving man. As they had no food or medicine to give him, one of the daughters, whose infant had recently died, nursed him. In *Roman Charity*, a painting in the Museum of Art in Puerto Rico, a woman is depicted feeding her imprisoned father, who had been sentenced to death by starvation (Figure 2.9). The daughter came to visit every day and breastfed her father through his prison cell bars. When this was found out, the Emperor, impressed at this familial dedication, released the father. The great Duke of Alva is said to have had two wet nurses in his old age, and the rich industrialist John D. Rockefeller reputedly drank nothing else in his golden years (a tidbit found noteworthy by Ripley's *Believe-It-or-Not*).

THE HEALING QUALITIES OF BREASTMILK

Breastmilk has been considered an especially valuable fluid for more than its use as a food source. In France, milk was as much a cosmetic as a food, at least among the ruling classes. The Roman Pliny gave this account:

Milk is valued for giving a part of its whiteness to the skin of women. Poppea, wife of Domitius Nero, took 500 nursing asses everywhere in her traveling party, and soaked herself completely in a bath of this milk, in the belief that it would make her skin more supple.

Figure 2.8
Women Breastfed the Aged

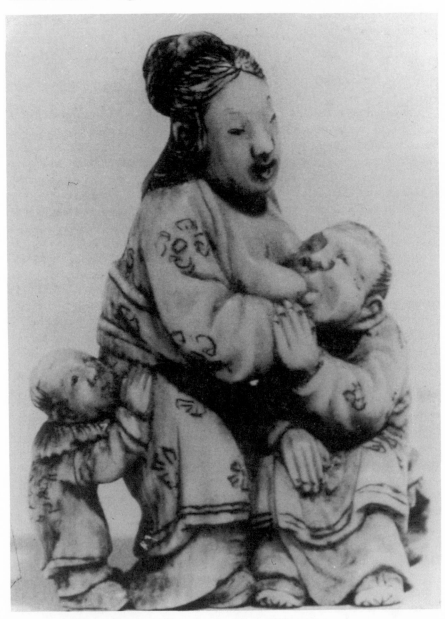

This *netsuke* (Japanese ivory figure) is a woman nursing her toothless great-grandaunt. The practice was used to keep her from starving. The elderly recognized the value of breastmilk and were often kept alive by their daughters or daughters-in-law at the expense of their grandchildren. *Source*: Staatliches Museum fur Volkerkunde, Berlin in H. Speert, *Iconographia Gyniatria* (Philadelphia: F.A. Davies Company, 1945). *Photo courtesy*: History of Medicine Division, National Library of Medicine, Bethesda, Maryland.

Figure 2.9
Roman Charity

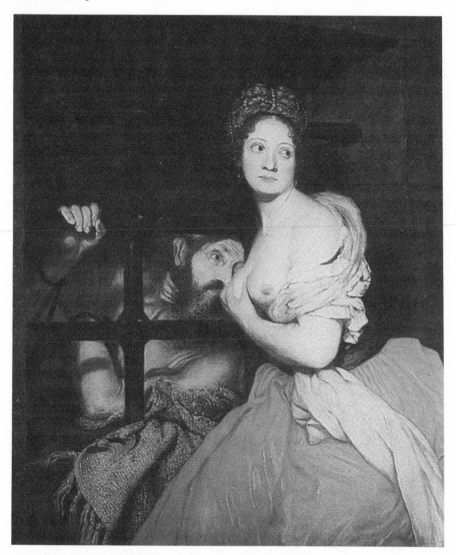

A daughter breastfed her father when he was imprisoned and sentenced to starve to death. When the Emperor discovered his secret to life, he was so moved by the daughter's dedication, he freed the father. Painting by Guido Cagnacci. *Photo courtesy*: Museo de Arte de Ponce, Luis A. Ferre Foundation, Inc., Puerto Rico.

Human breastmilk has a long history in medical therapeutics, particularly for treating disorders of the human eye. In the Egyptian medical document the *Ebers Papyrus* (1500 BC), breastmilk was prescribed for treating a variety of eye infections as well as being used to make a lotion for improving sight. "The milk of a woman who had borne a son" was an ingredient called for in several recipes for preparations used in the treatment of eye problems. One prescription used the milk of a woman who had borne a son "to drive out blood from the eyes" in combination with the fruit of the dom palm. Human milk has been used as a cathartic, for "sabs of the limbs" and for "uha-disease" (hookworm). As early as the eleventh century AD in Baghdad, Ali ibn Isa described human milk used in the treatment of eye diseases, including *ophthalmia neonatorum.*

Ancient Indians used breastmilk in eye operations and as a remedy for both eye and ear infections. It was also used as an antidote for opium intoxication. The uses were many, including "evacuating blood from the uterus"—wool soaked in breastmilk was inserted into the vagina. According to Pliny, women's milk was useful for fevers, feeble stomachs, pimples, spots, freckles of the face, and disease of the ears. The Chinese, too, were aware of the anti-infective properties of breastmilk. Among the twenty-four Chinese filial duties, one involved the son risking his life to get fresh deer's milk to cure his old parents' sick eyes.

In Samoa, when there was an epidemic of hemorrhagic conjunctivitis, breastmilk was squirted into the eyes of the affected patients when the supply of sulphonamides ran out. The Centers for Disease Control, in 1982, published the successful results of this old folk remedy.

The uses and permutations of breastfeeding are more widespread and more varied than most people realize. Few associate breastmilk with anything more than a mother quietly feeding her own child, if she chooses to nurse rather than use formula. Yet cultures around the world have found elaborate and extraordinary ways to use breastmilk to meet their goals—whether the goal was infant survival, maternal freedom, increased contraceptive protection, concern for the human infirm or aged, concern for the young of another species, or a pharmacological remedy. While modern societies focus on developing artificial replacements for breastmilk, past societies focused on developing clever and unique ways to take advantage of this marvelous fluid.

Most recently IgA deficiency in liver transplant recipients has been treated with human breastmilk. Mothers milk is a rich source of IgA which is protective against enteric infections and microbial translocation. Preliminary results in IgA deficient liver transplant patients indicates postoperative complications were lowered when patients were given breastmilk. (Merhav H.J., Wright H., Mieles L.A. and Van Thiel D.H. 1995)

Section II

Breastmilk: The Miracle Food and Medicine

Three

Cow's Milk Is for Cows

> The mammary gland in its perfected state, uninfluenced by disease or nervous disturbance or by the improper living of its owner, is a beautifully adapted piece of mechanism constructed for the elaboration and secretion of an animal food. When in equilibrium it represents the highest type of a living machine adapted for a special purpose, both mechanically, chemically, physiologically and economically.
>
> —Thomas Morgan Rotch, *The Hygienic and Medical Treatment of Children*, 1895

Breastmilk is inimitable. The alchemists of yesteryear promised they could transform rocks into gold; nowadays, chemists try to make artificial milk as good as genuine mother's milk. But just as the alchemists' efforts proved disappointing, synthetic milk substitutes have often proved unsuitable, sometimes even proved to be disastrous, and still do not have anti-infective properties despite efforts to "humanize" cow's milk. A plethora of research has demonstrated some of the incredible wonders of breastmilk and can only hint at potential new marvels as yet undocumented.

BREASTMILK IS SPECIES SPECIFIC

Biologically, breastmilk is highly complex and unique. It contains over one hundred constituents, each chemically different from the equally complex milks produced by other species. In the 1980s, well over 1,000 scientific papers were published on the biochemical properties of human milk, and yet recent findings (such as new polysaccharides found in breastmilk; the presence of an amino acid, taurine; and the increased bioavailability of iron and zinc) indicate that our base of knowledge is still incomplete.

Table 3.1
The Composition of Milks Obtained from Different Mammals and the Growth Rate of
Their Offspring

Species	Days to Double Birth Weight	Percent Content of Milk		
		Fat	*Protein*	*Lactose*
Human	180	3.8	0.9	7.0
Horse	60	1.9	2.5	6.2
Cow	47	3.7	3.4	4.6
Reindeer	30	16.9	11.5	2.8
Goat	19	4.5	2.9	4.1
Sheep	10	7.4	5.5	4.8

Source: L. Hambreus, *Pediatric Clinics of North America* (Philadelphia: W. B. Saunders Co.,
    1977) 24:17.

Each species of mammal has developed its own unique milk, chemically
superior for the offspring of that particular species (Table 3.1). Chemical
differences between species had been suspected for a long time. In the late
eighteenth century, scientific confirmation of these differences was clearly
established in the medical literature. In 1799, a physician named Michael
Underwood, on the fly page of his text, *Treatise on Diseases of Children*,
included a table comparing the differences in the milk of women, cows,
goats, sheep, and mares. This table served to highlight some of the obvious
differences and demonstrated that, of the milks that were examined, the
milk of mares was closest chemically to human breastmilk.

Although there are sharp differences in the composition of milk among
species, one important feature of all nonhuman mammals is that they suckle
their young until their babies can forage for themselves. Breastfeeding is
the crucial bridge between being in utero and being able to explore the
world on one's own. Just as the rate of growth and development varies
between mammals, so too is the nutrient composition of the milk species-
specific.

All breastmilks basically comprise the same types of substances, namely:
water, proteins, fats, carbohydrates, minerals, vitamins, cellular content,
and anti-infective agents. The quantity of each component, as well as the
quality of the nutrients, are linked to the digestion and absorption mechanisms of each species and are most likely determined by a genetic blue-
print. For instance, human milk has fewer salts than cow's milk, but the
salts are better adapted to a human infant's growth and metabolism (Table
3.2). Human milk has a small proportion of the volatile fatty acids that

Table 3.2
Comparison of Human Milk to Cow's Milk

Component	Human	Cow
Bacterial contamination	None	Likely
Anti-infective substances	Antibodies	Not active
	Leucocytes	
	Lactoferrin	Not present
	Bifidus factor	
Protein		
Total	1.0%	4.0% (too much)
Casein	0.5%	3.0% (too much)
Lactalbumin	0.5%	0.5%
Amino Acids		
Cystine/Taurine	Enough for growing brain	Not enough
Fat		
Total	4.0% (average)	4.0%
Saturation of fatty acids	Enough unsaturated	Too much saturated
Linoleic acid (essential)	Enough for growing brain	Not enough
Cholesterol	Enough	Not enough
Lipase to digest fat	Present	None
Lactose (sugar)	7.0% (enough)	3.0–4.0% (not enough)
Salts (mEq/l)		
Sodium	6.5 (correct amount)	25 (too much)
Chloride	12 (correct amount)	29 (too much)
Potassium	14 (correct amount)	29 (too much)
Minerals (mg/l)		
Calcium	350 (correct amount)	1,400 (too much)
Phosphate	150 (correct amount)	900 (too much)
Iron	Small amount	Small amount
	Well absorbed	Poorly absorbed
	Enough	Not enough
Vitamins	Enough	May not be enough
Water	Enough	Extra needed
	No extra needed	

Source: F. Savage King, *Helping Mothers to Breastfeed*, African Medical and Research Foundation, (*Nairobi, Kenya*: 1993).

cause indigestion; cow's milk has a large proportion of these acids. Not only does the amount of total protein between human and cow's milk differ (cow's milk has more than three times the protein of human milk), but the amino acid mix (amino acids are the building blocks of protein) is also significantly different. This has important implications, for example, in the development of the nervous system. Similar differences apply to most of the constituents of milk. In addition to the amount of each individual component, how readily it is absorbed also varies. Cow's milk contains more iron than human milk, but the iron in human milk has a higher rate of bioavailability; that is, the breastfed human infant absorbs more iron than infant fed cow's milk (49% compared to 10%). In fact, the newborn can absorb five times as much iron from human breastmilk as it can from cow's milk.

Although it has been known for centuries that asses' and goats' milks are actually closer in composition to human breastmilk than cow's milk, cow's milk has consistently been used as the primary human milk substitute. Decisions as crucial as these are not made based on nutritional superiority, but on economics. As anyone who has ever tried to milk an ass can attest, the task is near impossible. Cow's milk, on the other hand, is (and always has been) the easiest and least expensive milk to procure.

Not surprisingly, there appears to be a relationship between the composition of the milk and the survival of the species. Whale's milk, for example, has a high percentage of fat, a fact that allows the baby whale to quickly form a thick layer of blubber to protect it from the cold. The milk of the northern fur seal is 65% fat, also necessary for the seal young to form a thick coat of blubber as protection against the cold. The composition of the milk is also related to the rate of growth of a species. Where milk protein is high, the rate of growth is rapid. Humans are among the slowest growing of all the mammals. Calves grow at twice the rate of baby humans; baby rabbits double their birth weight in only six days. Rabbit milk is 14% protein, human milk is only 1.5%. Breastfed human infants are not expected to double their birth weight for four and a half months.

Breastfeeding has important implications for the survival of our species. Even today, in most of the world, breastfeeding is the single largest determinant of whether an infant lives or dies. One public health expert estimated that if breastfeeding were fully reinstated in developing countries, ten million children could be saved from diarrheal disease and malnutrition each year. If every newborn in the United States were breastfed for just twelve weeks, the health care savings from avoiding nonchronic diseases in babies' first year of life would amount to $2–4 billion annually. And the actual savings would be much greater, as breastfeeding confers a host of long-term health advantages (e.g., reduced incidence of allergies, asthma, heart disease, juvenile diabetes, obesity, etc.). An analysis of costs incurred because of the expense of infant formula and the extra costs in health care that result from formula-related illnesses around the world indicates that universal breastfeeding could produce an estimated savings of over $333 billion annually.

THE BREASTS AND MILK PRODUCTION

One frequent fear of small-breasted women is that they'll never be able to breastfeed. In fact, the size of the breasts has nothing to do with the quality or quantity of breastmilk. Large breasts contain more fatty tissue, not more milk ducts. A woman with small breasts can lactate just as readily as her buxom counterpart. It is the frequency of sucking and the ability of the mother to eject the milk through the let-down reflex that is critical to successful breastfeeding.

Breasts produce milk on demand. The mechanism by which this production occurs has intrigued humans for hundreds of centuries. Economists often joke that breasts represent the perfect system to exemplify the mechanisms of supply and demand. As long as a baby continues to ask for milk, the breasts continue to produce it. If the child stops asking (by ceasing to suck), the breasts stop producing. Technically, there is no such thing as empty lactating breasts.

Often thought of as mere blobs of fatty tissue, a woman's breasts are actually finely tuned chemical factories (Figure 3.1). The fantastic self-contained and self-regulated breastmilk factory is extraordinarily efficient. Its finely adjusted circuitry has at its core glands that release hormones on touch as well as in response to external stimuli received through nerve impulses. Heated sterile milk is manufactured within the breasts, then delivered promptly to the consumer directly through the glandular duct system. The fatty tissue of the breasts surrounds the glands and provides both protection and a source of energy (as well as giving the breasts their shape).

During pregnancy, about 3,000 calories worth of fatty tissue known as "lactation calories" are stored for lactation. Just as the fetus gets top nutritional priority when in the womb, from a breastfeeding point of view, the infant's survival also takes precedence. If the mother is malnourished or doesn't get enough calories when nursing, these fat reserves are called into use for milk production.

A woman's nipples are surrounded by nerve endings and blood vessels. When these nerve endings are stimulated (by touch, sucking, or even the sound of the baby crying), blood flows through the blood vessels and causes the nipples to become erect. Sucking also triggers the pituitary gland to produce the hormone prolactin. The nipple is surrounded by the areola, a circular pigmented area that contains large sweat and sebaceous glands. During pregnancy, oil glands (which appear as small bumps on the areola) enlarge and secrete sebum, which lubricates the areola and protects the

Figure 3.1
The Anatomical Structure of the Breast

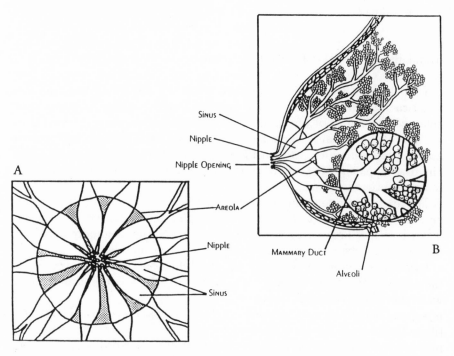

(A) Cross section of breast; (B) Structure of milk ducts. Diagrams by Barbara Heiser, RN, IBCLC.

nipple while the infant nurses. Within each breast are thousands of tiny cells, called alveoli, that produce milk when stimulated by the hormone prolactin. These tiny cells absorb water, salts, sugar, fats, and small nitrogen-containing molecules from the blood to create milk in milk sacs. There are between 2,000 and 16,000 milk sacs in each breast. The milk is delivered to the nipple through an intricate network of collecting tubes that join to become ducts, referred to as lactiferous ducts. There are fifteen to twenty ducts in each breast. As the sterile milk passes into the duct system (which is not sterile), the nipple picks up small amounts of microorganisms. Exposure to such organisms in these small quantities helps a child to slowly build up immunity to the organisms present in the environment.

Directly behind the areola are milk reservoirs, which serve as storage pools for milk left in the breast after a feed. The milk that collects in the ducts between feeds is called foremilk. When the infant begins to feed again, the foremilk is directed from these reservoirs into the baby's mouth.

Foremilk is high in protein but low in fat and calories, containing only fifteen calories per ounce. Hindmilk, the milk that is ejected from the mammary gland after let-down, is higher in nutrients and calories, containing twenty to twenty-five calories per ounce. It is essential that the baby receive a good balance of both foremilk and hindmilk. Hindmilk flows as a result of the ejection reflex that occurs when the pituitary gland releases the hormones prolactin and oxytocin when the nerve endings in the breast are stimulated by sucking. Prolactin stimulates milk production; oxytocin acts on the ducts to force the milk out. Anxiety, fear, pain, distraction, or stress can block this circuit. Drugs, too, can affect the delivery of milk. Pitocin (used to induce labor) and ergot (used to control uterine bleeding after delivery) can both act on the ducts to effectively block milk production.

The milk production system is self-contained and there is no need to prepare, clean, toughen, or soften the nipples in order to breastfeed. Rubbing the nipples with a coarse washcloth or applying lanolin or other oils is unnecessary even though many books and hospital staff often advise doing so. Cleaning the nipples with alcohol (which used to be a common practice) not only wipes away the natural lubricant, but also eliminates the distinctive specific odor of the sebum, which appears to be important for ensuring successful breastfeeding.

In a study conducted on weanling rat pups, three researchers examined the sensory aspects of suckling behavior. They found that when nipples were thoroughly cleaned, suckling was disrupted. Sterilizing the nipples interfered with the pups' desire to attach to the breast; returning the distillate of the wash extract back to the nipple reinstated attachment at normal levels. Thus, olfactory stimuli (smell) from the sebum is the major factor in nipple attachment. Mothers who sleep with their infants often notice that their newborns squirm right up to the nipple without opening their eyes; they do this by following the direction of the smell.

When applied to breastfeeding, preoccupation with sterility, often seen in hospitals around the world, may be counterproductive. In a nursery for premature babies in rural Africa, mothers were instructed to wash their breasts with cold water before feeding using nontouch techniques (in this case, by dangling their breasts under the faucet). Cold also inhibits the let-down reflex. It is easy to guess what happened to the breastfeeding rate. When looking at preventing the spread of disease, it is far more important for a mother to wash her hands than her nipples.

Breastfeeding is an interactive process between the baby and the mother. The act of the baby sucking is integral to the process. In fact, a "good milker" is a better description for a baby rather than a mother; if there is a problem with breastfeeding, it usually lies in the infant needing to develop a good strong sucking ability. One of the problems with bottle-feeding is that the liquid comes out quickly and easily and has a static consistency. Breastfed babies have to work for their milk; bottles deliver the goods so easily, babies feel full before their oral and touching needs are satisfied. This is why bottle-fed babies are much more likely to suck their thumbs and want pacifiers. Many anthropologists have noted the lack of thumb or object sucking in societies where prolonged breastfeeding is universal.

As long as sucking is sustained, the breasts continue producing milk. While milk production almost always is initiated through reproduction, the milk producing system is not dependent on reproductive function. Women can produce breastmilk without ever becoming pregnant (see chapter 2 for more information on this). Similarly, the breasts continue making milk as long as they are stimulated. Many a wet nurse breastfed for decades, even beyond menopause. In traditional societies, there are women who produce milk continuously; they are referred to as permanent lactaters.

Newborns are often born with the same hormonal influences that affect their mothers. Just as little girls sometimes have miniperiods shortly after birth, the pregnancy hormones produced by the placenta to prepare the mother's breasts for lactation also stimulate the infant's mammary glands. At the time of birth, infants (boys as well as girls) are actually equipped with developed milk ducts. After birth, milk (known as "witch's hazel") may even be found in the breasts of the newborns. If left alone, after a few days the infants' mammary buds dry up until shortly before puberty, when hormones once again appear to stimulate growth of the milk ducts.

BREASTMILK IS ALIVE

Colostrum is the first milk produced at the onset of breastfeeding. It does not look like milk. Referred to as "liquid gold," colostrum is a yellow sticky substance, rich in antibodies and high in protein, white blood cells, carotene, Vitamins A, B12, D, E, and zinc. It is produced in small quantities prior to the actual milk. In the first three to four days after the birth, the colostrum appears then changes to transitional milk; this in turn finally becomes the mature milk that will be sustained throughout the nursing period. When one talks of breastmilk, it is the mature milk to which one usually refers. Colostrum contains many of the same antibodies and nutrients found in mature milk, but in a very concentrated form, making it the ultimate food at a time when the baby is extremely vulnerable yet has low caloric needs.

Colostrum is produced by the glandular tissue in the breasts long before the baby is born. It is increasingly being recognized as vitally important to infant survival. In addition to its wondrous anti-infective qualities, it loosens extra mucus babies have at birth and also acts as a laxative to help to clear the digestive track of meconium (the first feces), which lessens the incidence and severity of jaundice. Colostrum is lower in fat and lactose and, as such, has fewer calories than mature milk (67 calories per 100 ml vs. 75 per 100 ml for mature milk). Generally, each feed provides the baby with about two teaspoons of colostrum. By contrast, most babies are drinking from twenty-eight to thirty-two ounces of milk per day by the time they are two weeks old.

During the first few days, mother and infant start getting to know one another. The mom gets accustomed to breastfeeding and the infant ingests colostrum. It is expected that breastfed infants will lose some weight as they build up their antibodies, because the nutrient density of colostrum and transitional milk is low. Babies may lose about 10% of their birth weight in the first few days while feeding on colostrum. Once the transitional milk comes in, the babies start gaining weight. Hospitals (concerned about weight loss) typically start all babies on formula immediately after the birth and/or give them bottles of sugar water, practices that are totally unnecessary and may be harmful.

Due to the imprecise definitions of breastfeeding, there have been a number of seemingly contradictory studies in the medical literature. The U.S. government's Women, Infants, and Children (WIC) Program, for instance, defines a breastfed infant as one who is nursed at least once a day. An infant can consume several pints of formula each day and still be categorized as breastfed. Others use vague terms such as partial, fully, or quasi-exclusive, which adds to the confusion.

The definition of exclusive breastfeeding is:

- breastmilk only (no water, juice, semisolids, or solids)
- initiation of breastfeeding within one hour of birth
- colostrum provided to infant
- infant fed on demand
- infant fed frequently (frequency of thirteen times per day in the newborn and less as breastfeeding is established and the infant grows older) (six or more times in twenty-four hours, including during night)

The problems created from the lack of precise definitions of breastfeeding are many. One study conducted in a Lahore, Pakistan, slum illustrates this point. When the research results were analyzed, it appeared that breastfeeding was not protective against diarrhea. When the information was reexamined, using a more accurate definition of exclusive breastfeeding, it was found that the infants who were nursed demonstrated significant protection against diarrhea.

Research has shown that exclusively breastfed babies are less likely to get infections, especially those of gastroenteritis (Figure 3.2), the respiratory tract, and the middle ear, and have significantly fewer allergies, with the most optimal effects achieved in exclusively breastfed infants.

One British study found that bottle-fed infants were forty-seven times more likely to be hospitalized for gastroenteritis than breastfed infants. Not

Figure 3.2
Relative Risk for Mortality Due to Diarrhea by Feeding Mode in Porto Alegre and
Pelotas, Brazil (Infants Ages 0–12 Months)

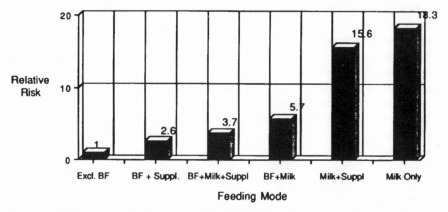

Source: C. Victora et al. *Lancet* 1, 319, 1987. *Graph courtesy*: Center to Prevent
Childhood Malnutrition.

only does breastmilk contain special anti-infection agents, but it is also ripe
with antibodies that coat the gut lining, protecting the newborn from germs
and also from the absorption of proteins that might cause allergies. Allergies are seven times less common in breastfed infants than in infants fed
on cow's milk preparations. Breastmilk protects us in ways we may never
fully understand. Interestingly, the success of kidney transplants is dramatically and significantly improved if the patient was breastfed, and the
chances for success are even better if the donor kidney came from a breastfed sibling.

Not only are breastfed babies healthier, they are smarter. A number of
studies show a link between infants reared on breastmilk and an increased
intelligence, but those studies have always been dismissed on the grounds
that mothers who breastfeed either were more motivated or had bonded
better, so there was no way to separate the mothering contribution from
the intelligence scores. A new study from the University of Edinburgh compared IQ test scores of almost three hundred premature babies. The infants
were born too small to suck. Half received breastmilk through a tube, half
received formula through a tube. The children tested for IQ when they were
eight years old. After taking into account the mother's social and educational status, the researchers found that the children who had received
breastmilk scored significantly higher on IQ tests. The study is not definitive
proof, but it offers very strong evidence that an as-yet-unidentified substance in breastmilk affects mental development. Breastfeeding, and espe-

cially exclusive breastfeeding, has untold benefits. Some of the known ones are listed in Table 3.3.

Breastmilk is a dynamic fluid. The milk of mothers of full-term infants is different than the milk of mothers with premature infants. Not only does the chemical composition vary daily, but it changes during each feed; foremilk is different from hindmilk. It even changes to reflect the needs of the child. Formula, on the other hand, does not contain living cells, has no antibodies, and does not alter to accommodate to each baby's changing needs. Formula, when made as instructed, is standard in content, consistency, composition, and color, quite unlike breastmilk.

The "let-down reflex" (also called "the draught" or "milk-ejection reflex") feels as if someone just opened the milk supply "tap"—the breasts suddenly balloon with milk (Figure 3.3). "Let-down" is a key neuro-endocrine reflex that is responsible for the ejection of milk. When the baby sucks on the nipple, a nerve impulse travels to the mother's brain and is then transmitted to her pituitary gland (this gland, called the "master gland," controls hormone secretions that regulate, among other things, growth, reproduction, and various metabolic activities). In seconds, the hormone prolactin is released; this stimulates the cells lining the ducts of the breasts, and milk is secreted. It is a very sensitive reflex, easily inhibited by psychological factors, and can be turned on and off by how a woman feels. The reflex can be triggered by thinking fondly of the baby or hearing the baby cry. Similarly, it can be stymied by tension, stress, or anxiety.

Unlike the reflexes that *make* milk, the "let-down" reflex is that mechanism that *releases* the milk. It signals the body to eject the milk into the terminal lacteals. With a successful "let-down," 90% of the available milk in the breasts can be obtained by the baby in less than eight minutes.

The hindmilk is essential to the infant's nourishment. It contains four to five times more lipids, one and a half times more protein, and, by far, the greater percentage of nutrients. Babies who are given "timed" feeds by mothers attempting to feed by a schedule (or as directed by doctors, who think it will minimize wear and tear on the nipples) receive plenty of foremilk but are short-changed of the calorie-dense hindmilk. Such babies appear to be unhappy and hard to console, as they are still hungry. Breastfeeding failure rates are always much higher when the length of the feed is determined by anyone other than the infant.

Viewed over the entire lactation period, breastmilk is remarkably consistent in composition, but at any individual time, its composition may vary. This is because breastmilk is alive. Every drop contains living cells that are constantly altering to accommodate to the infant's changing needs. Breastmilk comes with its own regulating substances that not only raise the bioavailability of some nutrients when this is useful but also lowers them when it is dangerous. Breastmilk also provides continual protection of the child. The milk produces antibodies against whatever organisms the mother

Table 3.3
Breastfeeding Benefits for the Child

Breastfed babies:
- get sick less often and get illnesses that are less severe
- are hospitalized less often and have a lower rate of mortality
- have a lower risk of diarrheal disease
- have a lower incidence of gastrointestinal illness
- have a lower risk of urinary tract infections
- have a lower incidence of respiratory disease
- have a lower incidence of otitis media (ear infections)
- have a lower incidence of allergies
- have lower rates of obesity
- have a lower incidence of sudden infant death syndrome (SIDS)
- have fewer learning and behavior difficulties
- have better psychological development
- develop a more energy-efficient and rhythmically functioning nervous system
- have a lower rate of pneumonia, neonatal sepsis, and giardia infections
- are less likely to develop heart disease and cancer later in life

Breastfeeding:
- helps bond mother and child
- confers passive immunities
- is protective against measles and other communicable diseases
- provides optimal growth and neurological development
- prevents malocclusion/leads to better teeth and jaw development
- protects against hypothermia
- provides partial protection against necrotising enterocolitis
- provides major protection against bacteremia and meningitis
- reduces the incidence of childhood lymphoma
- enhances visual development
- provides protection against neonatal sepsis
- is less risky for premature babies and babies with low birth weight

Artificially fed babies:
- haver a higher risk of diarrhea and infection
- have an increased risk factor for juvenile diabetes
- may have impaired antibody response to vaccines
- experience apnea and bradycardia more frequently
- have a higher risk of inflammatory illness
- have a higher risk of celiac disease, Crohn's disease, ulcerative colitis, cholera, and neonatal hypocalcemic tetany
- have a higher risk of obesity

Figure 3.3
Milk Production and the "Let-Down Reflex"

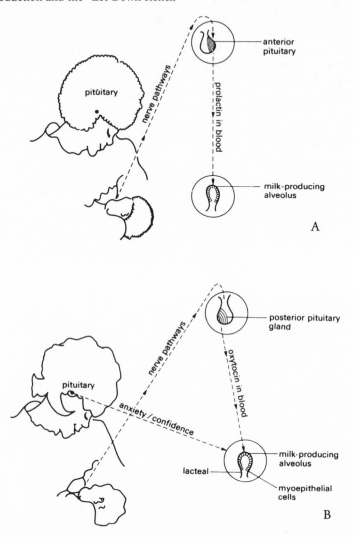

(A) The prolactin reflex (simplified); (B) The "let-down reflex" (simplified). Anxiety and confidence affect the "let-down" reflex (draught or milk-ejection reflex). *Drawings courtesy*: D.B. Jelliffe and E.F.P. Jelliffe, *Human Milk in the Modern World* (Oxford: Oxford University Press, 1978).

is exposed to, helping to protect the child from local pathological invaders. This ability of the milk to change both in response to the environment and to the child is part of the miracle of breastmilk. One mother may have chemically different milk than her neighbor, her sister, and a mother half-way around the world; however, except on rare occasions, any mother's breastmilk will be superior to any artificial food. This is why wet nurses and breastmilk banks have had such high success rates.

Chemists are not the only ones who appreciate the ways in which the breastmilk changes. The changes help breastfed infants control appetite and thirst. By choosing to stay on one breast for a long period and drinking the calorie-dense hindmilk, the infant's hunger needs are satisfied. By switching to the other breast and drinking the low-fat foremilk, the infant's thirst needs are satisfied. Having two breasts to draw from, one with whole milk and one with low-fat milk, gives the child the ability to meet both caloric and sucking needs.

The ability of the breastfed infant to regulate the caloric flow of milk may account for the different pattern of weight gain in breastfed and for-mula-fed infants. A World Health Organization (WHO) expert group is currently developing a growth chart for breastfed infants. The standard growth charts used by pediatricians today were derived from growth data on formula-fed infants. Not surprisingly, obesity is a greater problem with formula-fed infants than it is with breastfed ones. In one study, it was shown that only 19% of breastfed infants were obese, compared to 65% of bottle-fed infants (infant obesity is said to increase the risk of adult obesity more than threefold).

BREASTMILK COMPONENTS AND NIPPLE CONFUSION

Breastmilk is mostly water. In fact, human breastmilk is over 88% water. This is so for most mammals. Water serves the dual purposes of hydration and temperature regulation. Typically, as much as 25% of the body's water is lost daily through the skin and lungs from water evaporation (which is why water is so important). Breastmilk provides the baby with all the water needed, even in hot, humid environments. The soft stools of the breastfed infant indicate that water intake is adequate. Six to eight wet diapers in-dicate the infant has enough breastmilk.

A baby can become dehydrated easily, as its body has only a small amount of water. Breastfed infants are fed on demand, so they can hydrate themselves regularly. Studies undertaken in India and Honduras show that even in hot humid climates breastfed infants do not need to be given sup-plementary water. Formula-fed infants can only be fed every three hours, as that is how long it takes for an infant to digest artificial milk. Formula-fed infants living in hot environments do need extra water. In many hos-pitals, fear of dehydration leads staff to give water routinely to all infants. This practice has carried over to third-world countries, who often emulate "modern methods." Most hospitals use sterilized glucose water packaged in special bottles.

Diarrheal dehydration is the leading cause of infant mortality around the world because it depletes the infant of water and nutrients. When an infant develops diarrhea, water and solutes (in the correct proportion) are needed to prevent diarrheal dehydration and death. Plain water does not rehydrate the baby's cells or compensate for sodium loss, because the absorption of water is a complex process facilitated by certain salts and sugar. Special rehydration solutions are used (similar to athletes using "Gatorade" instead of water).

Infants get diarrhea from contaminated water or breastmilk substitutes. Health workers erroneously continue to instruct mothers to take the child off the breast if the child develops diarrhea. Breastfed infants with diarrhea should continue on breastmilk while receiving oral rehydration solution, whereas infants on formula must receive oral rehydration solution only. In addition to the use of oral rehydration solution for diarrhea, it has been found that time-tested folk remedies of rice water, chicken soup, or carrot soup are quite effective in restoring solute equilibrium and fluid repletion. Of course, breastfed infants under six months should not be given these. This is now called food-based rehydration and has an additional value of restoring nutritional status.

Not only is it unnecessary to give water to healthy breastfed infants, but it can be harmful when given in a bottle. The use of rubber nipples lessens a baby's instinctive efforts to open wide the mouth, conditions the infant to wait to suck until s/he feels the firm nipple in the mouth, and encourages sucking with the tongue pushed forward. These sucking techniques are exactly the opposite of what is required for breastfeeding (Figure 3.4). Infants accustomed to sucking on rubber nipples become easily frustrated with nursing, since milk from the breast does not flow as rapidly or easily.

The early introduction of bottles to breastfed infants or the use of mixed feeding interferes with the process of breastfeeding. It results in "nipple confusion," termed by Dr. Michael Latham as "the triple nipple syndrome" (Figure 3.5). Poor sucking technique can also result in trauma to the mother's nipples. Furthermore, an infant who nurses poorly because of incorrect positioning of the mouth and tongue will lose weight and, if the condition worsens, be labeled as a "failure to thrive." The mother will most certainly be told to give more formula, further undermining the breastfeeding effort. To help avoid nipple confusion, breastfeeding advocates also withhold pacifiers until breastfeeding is firmly established.

When this syndrome happens in developing countries, where it takes a small fortune to formula-feed an infant, mothers adulterate breastmilk substitutes by diluting formula or by adding sugar or oil to "stretch" it. Improperly prepared formula can result in malnutrition, illness, and even death.

Breastmilk content varies normally. The milk secreted will change slightly in color and composition throughout a feeding. While the color of formula

Figure 3.4
Nipple Confusion

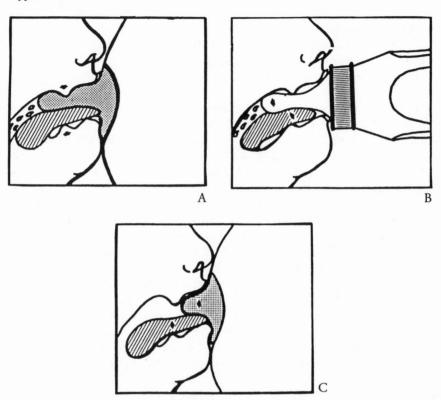

Sucking the breast and sucking the bottle require different actions. (A) Correct nipple and tongue placement during breastfeeding. Nipple and areola are well into the baby's mouth. The jaws compress the areola, and the tongue through peristaltic motions milks the breast; (B) Correct bottle feeding: The jaw does not need to compress bottle nipple. Negative pressure is all that is needed; (C) Incorrect breast-feeding after the bottle is given. As the tongue searches for the bottle it can push the breast out of the mouth. *Drawing courtesy*: Barbara Heiser, RN, IBCLC.

is consistent and corresponds to its concentration, the color of breastmilk cannot be used to make any diagnosis of the quality of the milk. What is remarkable is that even though the milk is changing continuously in response to changes in the mother's diet, it does not vary dramatically in quantity or quality. While it is important for the mother to consume a healthy balanced diet including sufficient fluids—64 ounces is recommended—during the nursing period, generally even a mother who lives on junk foods can produce enough breastmilk (*her* health will suffer, not the

Figure 3.5
Insufficient Milk Cycle Caused by the "Triple Nipple Syndrome"

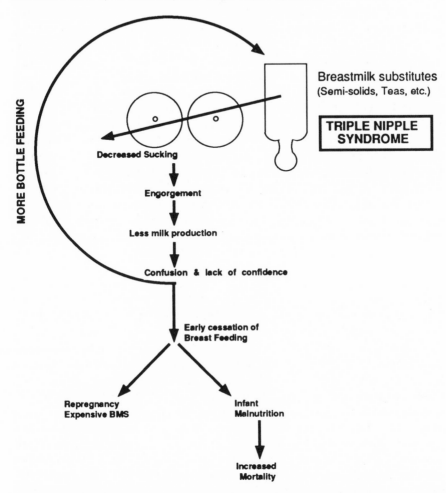

Nipple confusion results from mixed feeding. A vicious cycle is set up that affects the let-down reflex and milk production, resulting in the insufficient milk cycle. Once the cycle begins, cessation of breastfeeding is the typical result. *Source*: N. Baumslag, *Breastfeeding: The Passport to Life*. (New York: NGO Committee, Working Group on Nutrition, UNICEF, 1989).

baby's). A severely malnourished mother will produce less milk but enough to sustain healthy growth for a newborn for six months. Studies show infants can be successfully breastfed even under famine conditions. Most strikingly, even in conditions of severe starvation, where the amount of milk may be decreased, the quality remains remarkably constant. This is how infants are able to survive famines and wars.

Fat may be the scourge of nutritionists, but it is one of the vital substances that helps babies grow. Fully 30–35% of an infant's daily calories are supplied by milk fat. Consumers are used to selecting their supermarket milk by its fat content: nonfat, 1%, 2%, and regular 4%. Over the course of a day, babies have a similar variety of milk. Fat is the most variable constituent of breastmilk. Breastmilk contains up to 4.5% fat, but when and how much fat is delivered points again to the complexity of mammalian milk. The levels of fat in breastmilk vary with the time of sucking and the time of day. Not only is there a threefold increase in fat between the foremilk and the hindmilk; but also the fat levels change throughout the day, rising in early morning, leveling out about midday, then beginning to decrease again in the evening. The amount of fat in breastmilk is affected by both the diet of the mother and her nutritional status. Not surprisingly, malnourished women have a lower percentage of fat in their milk. The percentage of milk fat in any mother's milk is relatively constant over time (barring some dramatic change in her diet), dropping slowly the longer the duration of lactation.

Breastmilk also has higher levels of cholesterol than cow's milk. The exact significance of this is not yet known, but it may be an aid for early infant enzyme development. The exact make-up of fatty acids in breastmilk varies with the mother's diet. Cow's milk has more polyunsaturated than saturated fatty acids, whereas human milk has an almost equal quantity of each. Higher levels of polyunsaturated fatty acids, notably linoleic acid, are found in human breastmilk. The combination of fatty acids is important for infants; without it, skin lesions develop, growth is retarded or slowed, and wounds heal poorly. Breastmilk has 8–10% of its fat calories as linoleic acid; cow's milk has only 1.7%. (Interestingly, vegetarians have very high levels of linoleic acids in their milk.) Linoleic acid is important for nervous system tissue development. Serious problems arise in infants fed on cow's milk or formula without sufficient supplementation of linoleic acid. Another essential fatty acid found in breastmilk, called docasahexaenoic acid (DHA), is necessary for brain development and for visual acuity. It is not found in formula.

Protein is another important component of breastmilk. The proteins in milk consist of casein (curds) and lactalbumin (whey). The ratio of whey to curds is 1.5 in human milk, compared to 0.2 in cow's milk. There are twice as many curds in cow's milk as in human milk. On the other hand, whey levels are three times higher in human milk. These differences in milk protein composition are substantial. The lower amount of curd protein in human milk makes the milk easier to digest: it takes four hours for formula to be digested, only twenty minutes for breastmilk to be digested. The breastfed infant receives the bulk of its nutrients in just four minutes; not so with formula-fed babies. The infant's ability to digest breastmilk quickly is one of the reasons why breastfed infants can be fed on demand, while formula-fed infants are best kept on schedules of feedings no closer than four hours apart.

Like fat, protein has species-specific ingredients. Amino acids are the basic components that form protein. Cysteine, one of the essential amino acids, is present in human milk, whereas methionine is the primary essential amino acid in cow's milk. Human infants cannot metabolize methionine because the infant's liver in early life is immature. The amino acid, taurine, believed to be important for the development of the nervous system, is present in large amounts in human milk but wholly absent from cow's milk (it has recently been added to some formulas). Interestingly, very high taurine levels have been found in cat's milk. These amino acids are very specific, for example, kittens deprived of taurine develop damage to the retina resulting in blindness.

The whey proteins also differ among species in both composition and concentration. The chief constituents of human milk whey proteins are lactalbumin and lactoferrin, whereas in cow's milk the chief constituent is betalactoglobulin. The lacto-proteins make up the anti-infective part of milk that help the infant avoid disease. Lactoferrin is thought to protect the breastfed infant against certain gastrointestinal infections by binding the iron in these organisms and stopping their action. The current practice of giving newborns large doses of supplementary iron inhibits the lactoferrin, making it impossible for lactoferrin to do its job.

The predominant carbohydrate in breastmilk is milk sugar. The main sugar is lactose. Lactose is a disaccharide manufactured by the mammary glands from two monosaccharides, glucose and galactose. Even though the calories per ounce of breastmilk vary during a feeding, lactose is delivered in strikingly constant amounts (even when the volume of milk being produced is decreased, as in severely malnourished women). This sugar provides the infant with glucose and galactose, both of which are needed for the development of nerve tissue. Human milk has 6.8 grams of lactose per 100 ml, while cow's milk has only 4.9 grams per 100 ml. Lactose, as a sugar, not only provides an instant source of energy but is also important for the absorption of calcium.

Lactose is found only in mother's milk; it is not present in any other animal or plant source. This fact has led to the assumption that lactose may have a special significance not yet fully understood. (A few sea mammals, such as porpoises and dolphins, are the exception in that they have practically no lactose in their milk.) The enzyme (lactase) responsible for the digestion of lactose is found only in mammals, and while it is always present in the healthy full-term infant, it cannot be identified in a fetus before the thirtieth week of pregnancy. By the time a child is three years old, the enzyme has decreased, disappearing completely when the child is five.

It had been thought that if only small amounts of various nutrients were detectable in human breastmilk, breastmilk alone would leave the child necessarily deficient of certain growth factors. Nutrient studies have since shown that quality must be looked at in addition to quantity—and that looking at the concentration of specific nutrients alone is insufficient. The absorption of elements from human milk is much more efficient than either from cow's milk or formula. For example, studies have shown that whereas 49% of the iron in human milk is absorbed, less than 10% of the iron in cow's milk and only 4% of the iron in iron-fortified formula is absorbed. Iron absorption in formula declines with concentration. Some infant formulas contain twenty times more iron than breastmilk. There is a danger that this may affect the infant's response to infections by suppressing lactoferrin.

Breastmilk has enough iron available to prevent anemia in an exclusively breastfed infant. Ironically, the consumer willingly pays for an iron-fortified formula to ensure their child is getting this important mineral, yet the extra iron actually adds little value to the product. Most mammals have low iron levels in their milk, suggesting that absorption in the newborn is usually quite high. There still is controversy as to exactly how much iron an infant actually needs. As stated above, iron supplementation given to breastfed infants knocks out lactoferrin, a protective factor against gastrointestinal disease. Since the body is able to store iron, it is more appropriate to give iron supplementation to the mother in pregnancy, so that the infant can store sufficient amounts to get through the early months. Neonates' iron can be raised significantly by keeping the umbilical cord intact until after delivery of the placenta, waiting for the cord to stop pulsating and letting the blood drain back into the infant by gravity before severing the cord. By preventing the loss of 100 ml of blood, 45 mg of iron can be saved— more iron than one can get from formula in six months.

Zinc absorption from human milk also appears to be more efficient than from cow's milk. Acrodermatitis enteropathica, a potentially fatal condition, is a rare genetic disease caused by zinc deficiency. It occurs only in formula-fed infants and can be cured with breastmilk and/or zinc supplementation.

Vitamin C is another example of how the mother's diet affects that of the infant. While most mammals make their own Vitamin C, human infants are dependent on their mothers to obtain it. Breastmilk levels of Vitamin C rise within thirty minutes of the mother consuming it. In humans, Vitamin C is not stored, and a daily intake is necessary. In many clinics, mothers are told to give their infants orange or tomato juice from four weeks on to ensure their Vitamin C intake but this is not good as it may introduce infections. It would be better for mother and infant if the mother was given the Vitamin C and she passed it on to the baby.

Vitamins A (prevents eye disease and lowers mortality) and E (which is required for muscle integrity and resistence of red blood cells to hemolysis) are also present in large amounts in human milk. Vitamin E is important is preventing hemorrhage in the newborn. Colostrum is rich in Vitamin E and provides five times the amount that bottle-fed infants typically obtain from formula. Folacin (folic acid), a part of the Vitamin B complex, is also an important, more easily absorbed vitamin present in human breastmilk. Shortage of folic acid is not uncommon in pregnancy and has been associated with morning sickness as well as a variety of newborn problems such as premature births, low birth weight, and neural tube defects. In infancy, deprivation of this essential vitamin can result in retarded growth and anemia. As we have learned, if the mother has an adequate diet, the breastmilk has enough folacin, and the folacin present is more easily absorbed than is that in formula or cow's milk.

There are only two nutrients, Vitamins D and K, whose adequacy in breastmilk has been questioned. Vitamin D, for bone formation, is now considered to be present in adequate amounts in breastmilk, and colostrum has a higher concentration of Vitamin D than does mature milk. Recent research has revealed that there are significant levels of Vitamin K (prevents bleeding) in both colostrum and early milk, and that the highest proportion is found in the hindmilk.

Generally, ample vitamins for the child are present in breastmilk, except in the cases where a mother is on an extremely restrictive diet during pregnancy. In one case, a woman ate a very limited zen diet during her pregnancy. Her infant developed a nervous system disorder and retarded growth, two problems that could have been avoided if someone had noticed how restrictive her diet was. When fully investigated, she was found to be deficient in Vitamin B12, as was her milk; not surprisingly, her child was also deficient in Vitamin B12. The mother who has enough food and a variety of foods in her diet during pregnancy and lactation is unlikely to need supplements for herself or her fetus and should not engage in restricting her diet for weight loss after delivery.

BREASTMILK AND THE PREMATURE INFANT

Breastmilk is the ideal food for babies, large or small, term or preterm. The milk of a mother who delivers early is chemically different than that of a mom who delivers her baby after a full forty-week gestation. Preemies mother's milk is tailored to her baby's stage and will add to its growth and development as nothing else will. The act of nursing, itself, may be more difficult for preemies, but whether the baby is able to breastfeed right away

Table 3.4
Premature Infants: Benefits Attributed to Breastfeeding

- Human milk is easier to digest and better tolerated because the proteins are completely broken down and absorbed.

- Human milk contains an enzyme, lipase, that facilitates the digestion of milk fat, an important source of energy for the baby's growth.

- Human milk contains defenses against infection; preterm milk contains more concentrated antibodies than full-term milk.

- Necrotising enterocolitis is twenty times more common in preterm, formula-fed infants.

- Preterm infants fed formula are at a higher risk for Respiratory Distress Syndrome (RDS) and retinopathy of prematurity, prevented by inositol, absent in many formulas.

- Bottle-fed preemies have a higher frequency of apnea and bradycardia, as they lack respiratory control and the ability to self-regulate rapid milk flow.

- Preterm infants have higher protein requirements than full-term infants; preterm milk has four times more nitrogen than full-term milk.

- Preterm milk contains 30% more fat than full-term milk, providing readily available energy.

- In a clinical trial, formula-fed premature infants had lower IQ scores than breastfed premature infants.

- Human milk contains a plethora of hormones and enzymes, including various growth factors that may be important to the maturation of the digestive and nervous systems.

- Preterm milk is more suited to the unique nutritional needs of the premature baby, because it is higher in certain nutrients, such as protein, sodium, iron, linoleic acid, and chloride.

- Breastfeeding brings mother and baby closer.

---

or is fed intravenously or by tube, the food should be breastmilk. The mother's own unprocessed, fresh milk is the best for her baby. Next best is the mother's own milk that has been frozen. Pasteurized donor milk can also be used as a supplement or substitute. Finally, there are also special formulas for premature infants. Some of the advantages that breastfeeding provides for the premature baby are listed in Table 3.4.

Formula provides nutrients in a standard, consistent mix. But low birth weight and premature infants have small stomachs and immature kidneys. While formula is standard, breastmilk is dynamic, being automatically biologically prepared for the stage of the infant's maturity. The nitrogen content of breastmilk in the mother with a premature infant is higher, so much so that the premature infant fed on mother's milk receives 20% more nitrogen than a full-term infant fed mother's milk. Formula manufacturers have gone to great lengths to develop special formulas suitable for premature babies; Mother Nature takes care of this possibility effortlessly.

Formula-fed preterm infants are at a higher risk for respiratory distress syndrome (RDS) and retinopathy of prematurity if their diet is not supplemented with inositol during the first week of life. Inositol is a component of membrane phospholipids and reduces the severity of RDS by enhancing the synthesis and secretion of surfactant in immature lung tissue. Inositol concentrations are high in breastmilk and highest in preterm colostrum. Many formulas lack inositol.

Nipple confusion can be a problem with preemies as they get old enough and strong enough to suckle. In Kenya, premature babies are fed by cup, rather than bottle. At Pume Hospital in Beijing, China, all preemies are spoon-fed. This not only removes the possibility of nipple confusion, it also ensures that each child is held often. If the baby's parents can be at the hospital for feedings, they can take over this function, giving them a chance to both feed and hold the baby. In any case, working with the hospital to alert them that rubber nipples may cause problems can help avert difficulties down the road.

The mother who delivers early may doubt her ability to breastfeed and may have a baby too little to nurse, but both those obstacles can be overcome. A premature baby does not mean the baby should not nurse, it only means that the close, nursing relationship may have to wait until the initial difficult period has passed, a process that will go better with breastmilk.

THE FIGHT AGAINST INFECTION

The protective, anti-infective component of breastmilk has been mentioned several times. It is unique and of primary importance. Species-specific protective factors are present in both colostrum and mature milk (Table 3.5). Antibodies and other vital factors, such as lactoferrin and lysozyme, help the baby ward off invading disease organisms. Antibodies, such as immunoglobulin A (IgA), inhibit the growth of the dreaded diarrheal organisms *E. coli*, staphylococcus, and some fungi. A bifidus factor keeps the bowel at the right acid level by producing acetic and lactic acids from the lactose.

In addition to these antibodies and special factors, and unlike formula, human breastmilk has living cells that can phagocytose ("eat") germs. Breastmilk is one of the few substances that can actually attack viruses. Recent research has demonstrated an amazingly efficient function of the immunoproteins: they can attack germs and also be ingested as nutrient protein. The antibodies double as food supplements. Pathogens, such as the polio virus, are actually destroyed by antibodies in breastmilk and so are a wide range of organisms, including cholera, the giardia parasite, and certain fungal infections. This is one of the reasons why infants survive in impoverished, dirty environments.

Table 3.5
Anti-Infectious Factors in Human Milk

Bifidus
Secretory IgA and IgC
Antistaphylococcus factor
Lactoferrin
Lactoperoxidase
Complement C3 C4
Interferon
Lysozyme
B12 binding protein
Lymphocytes
Macrophages

Recent research has revealed that the mother actually stores up an immunological memory of all the pathogens ingested during her life, a memory that is retained in specific B cells in the lymphoid tissue of the small intestine. During lactation, probably under the influence of the hormone prolactin, these B cells migrate through the blood to the mammary and salivary glands, where they become transformed into plasma cells (Figure 3.6). These plasma cells secrete immunoglobulin A into the breastmilk in large volumes. This immunoglobulin remains in the infant's gut, where it prevents organisms from attaching to the gut wall and creating an inflammation. The mother's body is constantly biopsying her environment through her mouth; when she swallows a pathogen that her B cells are familiar with, she starts excreting the appropriate neutralizing immunoglobulin in her milk.

Roger Short, an Australian breastfeeding expert, expands this pathogenic memory concept:

Many animals including the higher primates will lick the faeces of their infants during suckling, thereby biopsying their excreta for signs of pathogens. Although humans do not normally indulge in coprophagia [dung eating] because of our revulsion at the smell of our faeces, it seems significant that women universally find the smell of the faeces of exclusively breastfed babies not the least unpleasant. . . . [T]here is ample opportunity for the mother, albeit unknowingly, to swallow any pathogen that her baby may be excreting, and subsequently passively immunize the baby against the organism with a specific IgA excreted in her breastmilk.

There is no way that any manufacturing process could ever tailor-make a synthetic milk to meet the different immunological demands of each and every infant.

Figure 3.6
The Entero-Mammary Circulation

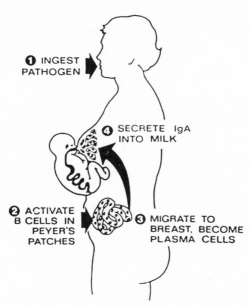

This illustration shows the protective action of breastmilk against gastroenteritis. *Source*: Roger Short, "Breastfeeding, Fertility and Population Growth," UNICEF, New York, 1993.

BREASTFEEDING BENEFITS FOR THE MOTHER

Most people have heard that breastfeeding is best for the infant, but are unaware that breastfeeding has life-saving benefits for the mother—both short and long term. Breastfeeding helps contract the uterus after childbirth, sheds the extra pounds of the pregnancy (a woman breastfeeding exclusively will burn 500–1,000 calories in one day), and helps the new mom feel relaxed and happy. Breastfeeding also protects the mother against diseases later in life. Women who have breastfed have lower rates of breast, ovarian, and uterine cancers, urinary tract infections, and osteoporosis (Table 3.6). It is nice to know that providing the best protection for the infant is good for the mother, too.

ISN'T FORMULA JUST A THIRD-WORLD ISSUE?

It has been long known that formula-fed babies are sicker, but it was assumed that the environment, not the formula, was the cause. Until the

Table 3.6
Breastfeeding Benefits for the Mother

- Bonds mother and child

- Provides the mother with a hormone-induced contentment

- Encourages efficient uterine contractions after childbirth

- Allows mothers to lose pregnancy weight and size faster

- Convenient (the milk is prewarmed, clean, and always available)

- Cost-effective and saves families money

- Contributes to natural family planning

- Contributes to household food security

- Fosters confidence and promotes self-esteem

- Reduces the incidence of urinary tract infections

- Protective against cancer (breast, ovarian, cervical)

- Lowers the incidence of chronic hepatitis

- Reduces the risk of hip fractures and osteoporosis

- Reduces the requirements of insulin for diabetic mothers

- Empowers the mother

- Gives her the right to choose

1980s, it was believed that the medical benefits of breastfeeding in modern, industrialized nations would be limited, as our generally high standard of living meant that bacterial contamination from the preparation and dispensation of formula would be minimal. It was presumed that where mothers could easily sterilize bottles and nipples, had ready access to clean water, and could afford appropriate amounts of formula, there would be no drawbacks to formula feeding.

In 1981, the U.S. government commissioned a task force to review the scientific evidence relating infant feeding practices to infant health. After studying the data, the task force concluded that breastfeeding prevented infantile gastrointestinal infections *in all settings*. Later research then determined that breastfeeding was associated with significant reductions in nongastrointestinal infections and with a reduced frequency of certain chronic diseases later in life. Not only was it confirmed that breastfed babies were healthier, but it was also found that the protection afforded by breastfeeding is greatest when bottle-feeding is excluded, and the protection declines in proportion to the degree of supplementation (with cow's milk or formula).

Yet, it is still widely believed that breastmilk confers health benefits only in developing countries, in spite of the overwhelming data published in the last ten years. It has been shown that in industrialized societies, a bottle-fed baby is five times more likely to contract gastrointestinal illness than is a breastfed one, *regardless of socioeconomic conditions.* Bottle-fed infants in the United States are hospitalized at a rate of up to twenty-five times higher than breastfed infants. One study analyzed hospitalization patterns for a homogeneous, middle-class, white, American population. Looking at the rates of infant hospitalization, it was estimated there would be seventy-seven hospital admissions for illness during the first four months of life for every 1,000 bottle-fed infants. The comparable figure for breastfed infants was five hospital admissions.

The UNICEF statistic that 1.5 million babies die each year because they are not breastfed applies to third-world babies. Most people assume that no child in the West dies because s/he is not breastfed, but a 1989 study conducted by the U.S. National Institute of Environmental Health Sciences estimated that four of every 1,000 infants born in the United States each year die because they are not breastfed. In 1992, 4.1 million American children were born. If half were bottle-fed (which is a conservative estimate), there would have been 8,168 unnecessary, preventable deaths.

In poor countries, diarrhea is the leading cause of infant death. While it is not the leading cause of death in the United States, five hundred children there, aged 1 month to 4 years, die each year from diarrhea. At least 70% of these deaths are caused by rotavirus infection, against which breastmilk has a known protective effect. Diarrhea in the United States costs over $75,000,000 a year for pediatric visits and $500,000,000 for hospitalizations.

Formula-feeding is considered a simple, safe, and sound practice. Yet even with clean water and adequate financial resources, breastfeeding is superior to artificial feeding in all places, at all times, and for all women.

THE BREASTS AND CONTRACEPTION

While women are suckling children menstruation does not occur according to nature, nor do they conceive; if they do conceive, the milk dries up. (Aristotle, 350 BC)

It is a well-known fact that, in the aggregate, exclusive breastfeeding is a potent contraceptive. Continued lactation brings with it the added benefit of suppressing ovulation. In cultures where women breastfeed their babies for long periods and use no artificial method of contraception, children are

Figure 3.7
The Contraceptive Effect of Breastfeeding

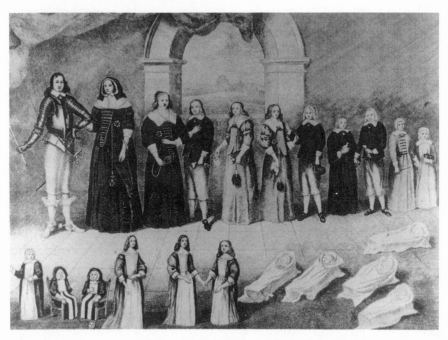

Seventeenth-century engraving of Sir Thomas and Lady Remmington of Lund,
Yorkshire, with their twenty children, five of whom died in childhood. Lady Remmington could never have produced so many children if she had breastfed them;
she most likely practiced the custom of the day of sending them out to be wet-
nursed. *Photo courtesy*: Roger Short.

spaced years apart. In cultures where mothers refrain from nursing, women
are often pregnant before the existing baby has cut a tooth (Figure 3.7). In
some countries today, breastfeeding provides more contraceptive protection
than all modern methods combined—and does so without taxing the
household's financial resources or endangering the woman's health.

Study after study has shown that breastfeeding is the single most effective
way of limiting conception in nations without access to birth control, that
is, in nations where frequent births spell frequent deaths. Children born
less than two years after their next older sibling are almost twice as likely
to die as those born more than two years apart. Spacing is the single most
important contributor to infant death. Promoting increased spacing can
prevent huge numbers—perhaps up to one-fifth—of these deaths, and a
considerable portion of maternal deaths.

While it cannot be said that any one individual woman will not ovulate while breastfeeding, it can be shown that a good many women do not ovulate the entire time they are producing breastmilk, or at least for the first year or more. The Kalahari !Kung bushwomen of Africa observe no sexual restrictions during lactation. The mothers nurse the babies for at least a few minutes several times an hour and sleep with their children. Births among the !Kung are spaced an average of forty-four months apart.

Individual hormonal levels, and perhaps individual nutrition levels, most likely determine the length of time of natural infertility. The key to limiting fertility appears to be the frequency of nursing, including giving night feeds. Using pacifiers, supplementing with formula, giving the child food when it requests the breast, or eliminating night feeds can result in a return of ovulation. Intervals of more than six hours between feedings and nursing fewer than five times a day can trigger the onset of fertility. One study of women who practiced total, unrestricted breastfeeding averaged 14.6 months before their periods returned. Nighttime feeding is essential to maintain the anovulatory state. Literature from formula companies has stressed the importance of getting a full night's sleep, without mentioning that infants obtain one-third of their nutrition from these nighttime feeds.

When menses have returned, a woman should consider herself fertile. Of course, ovulation can precede menstruation, so that a woman can be fertile a couple of weeks before her first postpartum period. However, in one study, only one-third of the women ovulated before their first menstrual period, and many of the first menstrual cycles did not contain sufficient hormone levels to support a pregnancy. Generally speaking, the longer the length of natural infertility, the greater the chances of ovulating before the first menstrual cycle.

A consensus statement on the use of breastfeeding as a family planning method was developed in 1988 at an international conference in Bellagio, Italy. The consensus of the expert group was that the "maximum spacing effect of breastfeeding is achieved when a mother fully or nearly fully breastfeeds and remains amenorrheic" (has no periods). When these two conditions are fulfilled, breastfeeding provides more than 98% protection against conception in the first six months. Following the Bellagio meeting, a program was developed to create a programmatic method of birth control using lactation. The Lactation Amenorrhea Method (LAM) adds structure and detail on how and when artificial methods of family planning should be provided. Lactation contraception should be augmented by artificial contraception when women start to menstruate, regular supplementation begins, or, for women who are breastfeeding exclusively, after six months.

Barrier methods of birth control are consistent with breastfeeding. Condoms, diaphragms, contraceptive sponges or foam, and cervical caps can be used with no deleterious effects. Oral contraceptives, including the new low-dose contraceptive pills, and any other method of birth control containing estrogen (such as the hormonal skin implants) should not be used by nursing mothers. They reduce the milk supply, alter the composition of the milk, and frequently lead to slower weight gain, the use of supplemental foods, and earlier cessation of breastfeeding. There is also concern that the contraceptive hormones can pass through the milk to the child. Long-term studies on this need to be done before conclusive evidence will be available.

IS MOTHER'S MILK ALWAYS SAFE?

In this age of alcohol, tobacco, and drug abuse; extensive use of agri-cultural and industrial chemicals; wide exposure to lead-contaminated soils, paints, and water; and new and fatal viruses, it is a concern to many that breastmilk may not be safe. The fear that breastmilk is a reservoir of con-centrated poisons is not new and is one more effort to discredit breastmilk. There has always been speculation that artificial feeding was a way of sav-ing children from their mother's contaminated milk.

Broad conclusions about potential contamination of breastmilk are hard to make. Not only does each case involve a wide array of factors from the diet of the mother to the air she breathes, many of the suspected toxins are new enough to preclude any long-term studies. Claims of contamination must be looked at in light of their source: environmentalists often exag-gerate the degree of contamination to boost their case for greater safe-guards, and formula companies freely spread fears of toxins in the hopes that mothers will choose formula as a way of erring on the side of safety. On the other hand, some breastfeeding promoters would have you believe that breastmilk is impervious to contamination.

When looking at any claims of breastmilk contamination, it is also im-portant to remember that any baby exposed to something through breast-milk was almost certainly exposed to the hazard during pregnancy. This means several things. First, an infant showing a higher than desired level of a toxin may be obtaining it from the breastmilk, but more likely it's from exposure in the pregnancy. Second, the presence of something in the breastmilk does not necessitate that the substance is harmful to the child; the role of milk contaminants in the production of disease in children is virtually unknown. Third, all discussions of breastmilk contamination have as an underlying assumption that formula is always clean and safe. As we will see later, this is not necessarily the case.

An environmental concern at issue is the chronic exposure of breastmilk to toxic fat-soluble chemicals. One of the functions of body fat is to remove toxins from the bloodstream and to store them. Women have long been warned to avoid crash diets during lactation. Not only are they a bad idea in general, but a sudden drop in calories triggers the body to use fat (re-ferred to as lactation calories), thereby potentially releasing toxins into the bloodstream and breastmilk. Fat-soluble chemicals accumulated in the woman's fat and subsequently released into her breastmilk may expose the infant to unacceptably high levels of specific toxins, leading to impairment of the brain's development, liver and kidney damage, as well as early cancers. The primary environmental culprits are chronic exposure to chlorinated chemicals (such as heptachlor), pesticides, and industrial poisons (such as PCBs and DDTs), dioxins (such as Agent Orange) and furans (solvents for resins and plastics), and heavy metals (such as mercury, arsenic, and lead). Exposure to these is generally in the form of food contamination from agricultural products and especially fish. However, to date, no human toxic effects have as yet been attributed to these substances, even when they have been found in breastmilk and exist in large amounts in the environment.

The presence of toxins in breastmilk could frighten mothers away from breastfeeding. However, the importance of breastmilk for optimal infant nutrition, as well as for providing antibodies, outweighs any potential danger of the contaminants. Only where there is heavy exposure to toxins is there a reason to consider breastfeeding alternatives. Recommendations for women to minimize chemical exposure include eating a varied diet, avoiding fish from contaminated waters (especially fish from the Great Lakes, polluted fresh water, and game fish), and not losing excessive amounts of weight. Chemical analyses of breastmilk contamination are difficult because breastmilk varies widely from woman to woman and changes considerably over the course of each feeding. Women who have eaten contaminated fish, who live near a waste disposal site or heavily industrialized area, or who have been involved in environmental spills should check with their midwife/ obstetrician or the Food and Drug Administration (FDA) for specific advice or testing (most large hospitals are equipped to test breastmilk for toxins or can arrange for a laboratory to do so).

Breastmilk may offer the most protection against some toxic chemicals. Information from Italy and Austria shows that breastmilk contained one/ three-hundredth the amount of radioactive iodine and caesium that was found in cow's milk following the Chernobyl accident. This was confirmed by Swedish studies. During this radioactive episode, all the cow's milk in a wide region had to be discarded. Resulting shortages of both fresh milk and infant formula put all artificially fed babies at risk. Additionally, the radiation levels in breastmilk were much lower than were the levels in the mother's body, leading researchers to conclude that some mechanism exists that reduces the radioactive materials in the milk as it is produced.

When there is concern about toxins in the breastmilk, it is also important to realize that there should be a concern for all of society, not just for pregnant women and nursing babies. The chemicals and toxins that we allow in our environment may affect breastmilk, but they also affect the fetus and are known to cause cancer, lead to learning disabilities, and wreak havoc on wildlife. Discussing breastmilk contamination is useful as a vehicle for promoting efforts directed at a cleaner environment, but obsessing over breastmilk contamination is harmful if it only serves to scare mothers while ignoring the larger issue of contaminating the planet.

Almost everything that a woman ingests affects her breastmilk. This includes nicotine, caffeine, alcohol, and drugs. Some of these substances can be found in breastmilk as soon as thirty minutes after consumption. With most potentially problematic additives, the effects on the baby are directly related to the quantity of the substance the mother ingests. Moderate use of almost anything does not pose a threat to a child. Obviously, the better one's diet, the better it is for both mother and baby. People are not perfect, however, and many women, reticent to give up their lifestyle habits, abstain from breastfeeding because of fears that their milk is not good enough. In reality, the child is better off breastfeeding than receiving artificial foods. Most drugs are found in the milk, but the concentration is usually low enough that there is little likelihood of an effect on the infant. "Moderate" is considered to be up to two alcoholic drinks per day, no more than the amount of caffeine in five cups of coffee each day, limiting smoking to a pack of cigarettes a day, and minimal use of illicit drugs. The more a mother engages in activities that could be harmful to the infant, the more likely it is that breastmilk production will be affected adversely. The greater the threats to the child, in general, the greater the chances that the mother's body will shut down the breastmilk supply. Once this happens, the baby is in double jeopardy: first by facing potential inadequate nutrition, and second by having a mother possibly too impaired to properly care for the infant. The good news is that breastfeeding triggers the release of the hormone oxytocin, which has the effect of calming a mother and focusing her interest and attention on the baby. Because of this chemical involvement, the breastfeeding mother is more likely voluntarily to alter her detrimental habits than the formula-feeding mother.

There are various diseases that it is feared can be transmitted through breastmilk. Generally, the main route of transmission of infections is through skin contact and secretions from the nose and mouth, not through breastfeeding; thus good hygiene is the area where effort should be concentrated for disease prevention. Nursing through a cold, flu, or minor infection does not hurt a baby, and offers tremendous protection to the infant against these contagions. Women with fevers can similarly continue to breastfeed but should be careful to drink extra fluids to decrease the chances of becoming constipated and dehydrated. There is a lot of misinformation about breastfeeding and infections. This is particularly so with regard to breast infections. Mothers are told incorrectly to stop breastfeeding because the infection passes through the milk to the baby. The best treatment is to keep nursing, apply compresses, and use the prescribed antibiotic. Many babies have been taken off the breast unnecessarily when infections have developed. In terms of specific diseases, there is no evidence that cholera and typhoid fever are transmitted through breastfeeding. In fact, there is evidence that a mother exposed to either of these helps protect a baby from getting them. Women with hepatitis A who have no symptoms can breastfeed. Women with hepatitis B can have the child vaccinated so that breastfeeding can continue uninterrupted. There is no evidence that malaria or Lyme disease can be transmitted by breastfeeding. Breastfeeding can continue through most diagnostic tests, ultrasound, CT scanning, magnetic imagery, biopsies, and surgery. After a general anesthetic, a mother can nurse as soon as she is alert enough to handle her child. Medications that are compatible with breastfeeding can usually be found. Interestingly, in some chronic illnesses, such as rheumatoid arthritis, lupus, and multiple sclerosis, breastfeeding may give the mother a period of temporary remission.

Not every disease and treatment however is compatible with breastfeeding. Chemotherapy and treatments with radioactive compounds require weaning a child (if a radioactive iodine is used for diagnostic purposes, breastfeeding can resume after twenty-four hours). Food poisoning that becomes systemic requires an interruption of nursing. A herpes sore on the nipple or areola is sufficient cause to withhold the breast, although the mom can nurse on the uninfected breast (milk pumped from the infected breast should be discarded). Women suspected of having toxic shock syndrome may have toxins in their milk that could harm the baby.

With the increasing prevalence of HIV infection, more and more women of childbearing age are infected and therefore able to pass the infection on to their children. Roughly one-third of the babies born to HIV-infected mothers worldwide become infected themselves. Most of this transmission occurs during pregnancy and delivery. Data reported recently suggest a small number of babies have become infected through breastfeeding. To date, there have been no proven cases of HIV transmission from milk donated to a milk bank. (In fact, there have been more cases of HIV transmission from artificial insemination than suspected cases of transmission from breastmilk.)

The vast majority of infants breastfed by HIV-infected mothers do not become infected, but definitive answers to many questions are still lacking. The timing of HIV infection appears to be a crucial factor. The risk of HIV transmission is greatest when women become infected after they conceive and among those who seroconvert (switch from HIV-negative to HIV-positive) when they are pregnant or breastfeeding. This is thought to be due to the fact that when a person first contracts HIV or seroconverts, s/he may be briefly more infectious due to high virus levels in the blood and to antibodies not yet having developed.

Internationally renowned experts from the Centers for Disease Control (CDC), WHO, and UNICEF have devised a two-tiered strategy to address the issue of whether HIV-positive women should breastfeed. They have concluded that where infectious diseases and malnutrition are the main cause of infant deaths, breastfeeding should be pursued because the baby's risk of HIV infection through breastmilk is likely to be lower than their risk of death from diarrhea dehydration if s/he is not breastfed. In places where the infant mortality rate is low and the main cause of infant deaths is not infectious diseases, such as in the United States, women with AIDS and those who are HIV-positive are being advised to use infant formula (though pasteurizing breastmilk is also known to be safe).

It is known that babies who are not breastfed are at higher risk of becoming ill and succumbing to infections. It is also known that breastfed babies who are HIV-positive develop AIDS later than children who are formula-fed. The evidence is unclear but may indicate that withholding breastmilk, with its impressive health-protecting factors, may actually increase the risk of children developing AIDS. Nutritional factors may also be important in the vertical transmission of AIDS. Vitamin A deficiency during pregnancy was associated with a three-fold to four-fold increased risk in mother-to-child transmission and a high perinatal and infant mortality (Semba et al., 1994).

The AIDS scare, in particular, has resulted in the hasty closure of many breastmilk banks, which may have led to preventable infant deaths. Blood banks entail a larger risk than do milk banks, but because blood is valued, precautionary measures have been taken such as asking high-risk groups not to donate and undertaking routine testing of blood. One reason breastmilk may be underappreciated is that it is generally donated, not sold. Blood is often bought, and a clear monetary value is associated with it. To date, there have been no reported cases of AIDS spread through donated milk.

It would be an overstatement to say that breastmilk should be used at all times and in all places, but it is not an overstatement to say that breastmilk should be used at almost all times and in almost all places. There are clearly times when withholding breastmilk is in the best interest of the child, but these times represent the exception, not the rule.

IS COW'S MILK ALWAYS SAFE?

Cow's milk, a common product in this country that has often been dubbed "nature's most perfect food," is not looking so perfect anymore. Milk was right up there with products that were as wholesome as apple pie, but no more. Concerns of milk safety have alarmed consumers, while the industry is worried as consumption goes down (as soft drink and bottled water consumption continues to increase) and government price supports continue to decline. Feeling under attack, the U.S. dairy industry has launched an aggressive and sophisticated marketing campaign to get consumers to consume more milk.

Dairy industry officials stress that no other food product is tested as often or as thoroughly as milk. From the cow to the consumer, milk is continually checked for temperature, bacteria, color, odor, added water, antibiotic residues, and a host of other factors. Yet concern about the safety of milk continues to be fueled by a number of studies. Studies have found that cow's milk can have extremely high levels of chemical and hormone residues. In fact, the levels of pesticides in human milk are typically less than those in cow's milk, since cows eat both plants and the dirt in which the plants are grown. In 1989, the *Wall Street Journal* found that 38% of fifty milk samples collected in ten cities around the country were tainted with antibiotics and sulfa drugs. The Center for Science in the Public Interest found in 1989 that four of twenty milk samples collected in the Washington, DC, metropolitan area contained residues.

Not only are things showing up in milk that aren't supposed to be there, but also things that are supposed to be there cannot be counted on. A recent spate of illnesses in Massachusetts unveiled a problem with the levels of Vitamin D fortification in milk. Scientists recently evaluated seventy-nine samples of milk from ten states: 80% contained 20% more or less Vitamin D than labels indicated, 14% had no detectable Vitamin D at all, and one container of milk contained 914% more than it should have. For infant formula, the likelihood that the Vitamin D content matches that described on its label is remote. When infant formulas were tested, most contained about twice as much, and some up to 4.5 times as much Vitamin D as labeled. Vitamin D is essential for the absorption of calcium (for bone formation) and to the function of muscle and many other tissues. For the population at large, varied Vitamin D levels do not present too much of a hazard, but for infants and the elderly, it can be serious. In the fall of 1990, doctors at Harvard became alarmed when a fifteen-month-old child and a seventy-two-year-old woman fell ill with Vitamin D intoxication. That same year, eight more people in Massachusetts became ill from excessive amounts of Vitamin D in milk. The milk they drank ranged from a Vitamin D content from near zero to more than 500 times the recommended amount. Toxic doses of Vitamin D cause convulsions and kidney damage due to hypercalcemia and may cause long-term mental consequences.

Concern over the safety of commercial cow's milk has been heightened by the controversy over Monsanto Company's controversial recombinant Bovine Growth Hormone (rBGH). Cows treated with rBGH produce 10–30% more milk than do standard cows. However, the additional lactation comes at a cost. rBGH-injected cows suffer from what is called a "prolonged negative energy balance." Known side-effects of the drug, according to the manufacturer, include reproductive problems (such as infertility, retained placenta, and cystic ovaries), mastitis and poor general health, increased heat stress, digestive and foot disorders, anemia, and sometimes severe injection-site reactions. The drug was recently approved by the FDA in spite of the facts that we don't need more milk (the U.S. government has spent $10.6 billion buying up surplus dairy products and continues to buy milk surpluses) and that the milk from hormone-treated cows has not been proven safe.

There are several health concerns associated with drinking this milk. One concern is that these cows are known to have more health problems (a 79% increase for clinical mastitis alone), which in turn leads to increased use of antibiotics, resulting in even more drug residues in milk. Another concern is the risk of breast cancer from the consumption of rBGH milk. Research has shown that rBGH in milk induces a sustained increase in Insulin Growth Factor (IGF-1), a growth factor for human breast cancer cells that helps them maintain their malignancy, progression, and invasiveness. *Newsweek* magazine has called rBGH "a medical disaster" in the making.

The rBGH controversy has brought local and national farm, environmental, consumer, and animal protection groups together to oppose rBGH and to push for mandatory labeling of products made from cows who have used the hormone. Parents in the school district in the town of Wisconsin Rapids, in a state where dairy cows are nearly sacred, were so upset about their children consuming rBGH-tainted milk that they convinced the district to offer elementary school children the option of juice instead of milk in school lunches. The Los Angeles school district has banned milk from rBGH cows. Land O' Lakes and Marigold Foods, two large milk-marketing companies, recently announced new brands of milk certified as coming from cows that haven't been treated with rBGH. More than one hundred food retailers and manufacturers, ranging from 7-Eleven stores to Ben & Jerry's Homemade Ice Cream, have announced that they will not sell dairy products from rBGH-injected cows.

The European Community has a moratorium on use of the hormone (even though it is made in Austria and packaged in the Netherlands, under the brand name POSILAC). Monsanto has already received licenses to sell rBGH in Brazil, Mexico, and South Africa. Field trials have begun in Argentina, China, Egypt, India, Malaysia, Pakistan, Tunisia, Zambia, and Zimbabwe. The hormone is illegal in New Zealand and Australia.

Milk has come a long way from its image as a wholesome, nutritious food source. As more and more adults abstain from drinking milk due to concerns about its safety, we should be asking if a product that isn't safe enough for adults is safe enough for children. Few women would choose to have themselves injected with an untested hormone to increase their milk supply if it would, in turn, give them mastitis and reproductive problems. Yet this is the milk that will be the basis of the majority of infant formulas and the product given to children when they no longer require formula.

IS FORMULA ALWAYS SAFE?

Hindsight shows the story of formula production to be a succession of errors. Each stumble is dealt with and heralded as yet another breakthrough, leading to further imbalances and then more modifications. (Dr. Derrick Jelliffe, *Wall Street Journal*, 1980)

As consumers increasingly worry about toxins from the body polluting the breastmilk, the prevalent notion is that substituting formula for breastmilk would assure a certain level of safety. However, formula is far from a reliably clean, pure product, and abandoning breastfeeding in response to toxin concerns may be self-defeating. Formula may contain even higher levels of toxins, specifically aluminum, lead, and iodine. Although they receive little adverse press, there are no shortages of instances when the formula on the store shelves has been anything but clean, safe, and pure. In the ten years from 1983 to 1993, formula was recalled twenty-two times due to safety problems, well over half from instances where the product would cause death or serious health consequences, in some cases, irreversible. Appendix C lists FDA recalls for the years 1982–94.

The composition of formula, a chemical preparation, is subject to human error. In 1992, the Consumer Council of India found live black insects and crawling worms in a 500 gram packet of Lactogen baby milk. But again, this is not just a third-world issue. In 1979 there was a problem with alkalosis caused by a batch of infant formula deficient in chloride. In 1985, deaths of two infants were reported who were diagnosed with aluminum intoxication from powdered formula. In 1986, a U.S. factory had to be shut down because persistent salmonella in the powdered baby milk could not be eliminated; in 1985, an infant had died from salmonella, the source powdered formula contaminated at the factory. In 1989, sepsis and meningitis were diagnosed in a handful of infants who received formula containing the bacterium *enterobacter sakazakii*. In 1990, 63,760 gallons of a liquid soy concentrated formula were recalled for contamination. FDA inspectors noticed the cans were swollen, some ready to burst. The company did not determine the source of the contamination, and a month later found that cans from an entire production run were starting to swell. The plant was shut down. Recalls for contamination have not stopped. Recalls are issued for a variety of reasons from contamination with bacteria (including salmonella) to cans containing broken glass bits.

Laws governing the manufacture of infant formula are minimal in scope. In 1980, U.S. law only dictated that formula must be manufactured under sanitary conditions and that the label must state the ingredients. The current law is only slightly better. Quality control is difficult to maintain even in ideal conditions.

In the United States, where a safe water supply is almost universally available, very few people question the role of the water used in preparing formula. But water used in the manufacture of baby formula as well as water added at home can be unsafe. For example, two brands of Abbott Laboratories formulas in the United States were found to contain several carcinogenic chemicals due to contaminated well water. "Blue Baby" syndrome is a risk for formula-fed babies from a high nitrate content in water, usually resulting from the leaching of artificial fertilizers. Nitrate levels in water must be regularly monitored and controlled. Water engineers also worry about other chemical residues in waters.

To compound matters, parents may inadvertently be turning perfectly safe formula into poison. Formula-fed infants are at a higher risk for ingestion of lead. This is frequently due to the practice of boiling the water used to mix the formula. Instructions of the label advise boiling water for five minutes before mixing; however, this action concentrates any lead in the water and dramatically raises the amount of lead in each feeding. But unboiled water is also risky in certain areas. During recent state-mandated screenings in Boston, pediatricians were alarmed to find a large number of infants with dangerously high lead levels in their blood. The lead source was from unboiled tap water used to make formula. Parents were using the first water out of the faucet in the morning (the first water flowing through the pipes contains the highest lead concentrations). Recommendations include having home water tested for lead levels; using bottled water if the level is high; or, if the levels are acceptable, letting the tap water run for at least two minutes before using it, boiling the water (if necessary) with a lid on the pot, and not using lead pots for boiling water.

Even when a perfectly safe can of formula is being used with perfectly safe water, there is still a further risk. If formula is not mixed as instructed on the label, it can cause serious health problems such as malnutrition, hypernatremia (too much sodium), and metabolic stress. As the price of formula has skyrocketed (see chapter 5) over the last ten years, there has been an epidemic of water-intoxicated infants seen in low-income populations. The inability to pay for sufficient formula is blamed for this. At the other extreme is a recent case from Buffalo, NY, where the mother lost the measuring scoop and guessed incorrectly at the proper proportions of formula to water. She gave the baby a superconcentrated solution that caused severe hypernatremia, convulsions, and death. Babysitters and grandparents often add an extra scoop or use a heaping scoop feeling that this will be a treat for the baby or that it will help the baby to sleep more soundly, cry less, grow faster, or make it happier. This is a dangerous practice.

Formula is a specific chemical composition designed to be carefully measured, prepared, and used in a specific way. Unfortunately, many consumers treat it more like powdered milk and assume that adding extra will simply make it richer and better, or that adding more water will make it last longer. Formula companies have not made consumers aware of the dangers of either underdiluting or overdiluting. In addition to better labeling, mixing instructions that use a common household measure should be provided so that the correct dosage can be mixed readily without having to locate a specific scoop.

Formula has the image of being safe, but unfortunately the product has a history of both documented and undocumented problems, including fatalities. Very few people worry, when they put the can of formula from the grocery store shelf into their shopping cart, if there will be glass particles in the powder, if it will be deficient in essential nutrients, or if the water they will be mixing it with will have high levels of lead, but these are real concerns, and pretending these dangers don't exist won't make them go away.

IS BOTTLED WATER ALWAYS SAFE?

Many women who bottle-feed their infants also supplement the baby's diet with bottles of commercially sold water. This is done for a number of reasons: the hospital staff gave the babies bottled water, so mothers assume it makes sense to do it at home; it gives the baby something to suck on between meals; it helps keep fluids in the body when it is hot or dry or the baby is congested; and it is an inexpensive product that is viewed by many as an adequate feeding supplement. Unfortunately, something that appears as innocuous as giving a baby bottled water can have serious consequences.

"Water intoxication" is the illness associated with feeding infants bottled water. It is characterized by an altered mental state, hypothermia, swelling, and seizures and is most commonly seen in infants less than six months old. Babies who experience water intoxication usually recover fully but usually require hospital admission and need intravenous solutions to adjust their salt levels. The condition was first reported in 1967 and is seen most commonly among infants of parents living in poverty. Poor parents are more likely to substitute water bottles for formula in an attempt to stretch out the costly cans of formula.

Bottled waters portray the image of purity and wholesomeness, but in some cases, tap water is a better choice because it has a greater number of minerals. The FDA has recommended to the International Bottled Water Association that the labels of commercially sold waters clearly indicate their content and appropriate uses (such as rehydrating infant formula and diluting juices), but that they not be used in lieu of infant formula. Several manufacturers have submitted their existing labels for FDA review. Breast-fed babies do not need any supplemental fluids, but in some cases formula-fed babies do. Parents and caretakers of formula-fed babies need to be educated about the potential hazards of feeding water to infants.

LACTATION-SUPPRESSING DRUGS

As America increasingly becomes a bottle-feeding culture, more and more women want to terminate lactation in the most efficient and effective manner. Women who choose to forgo breastfeeding altogether have two postpartum options: wait for their breastmilk to dry up (it takes about ten days) or take lactation-suppressing drugs. In an assumption that a few pills at the hospital are all that is needed to solve the lactation problem, many maternity patients opt for the drugs. Each year, 1.8 million new mothers in the United States elect not to breastfeed. About 800,000 of them are prescribed lactation-suppressing drugs.

Letting the breasts produce the milk then respond to the lack of sucking by curtailing the milk flow poses no risks to the new mother. It is not always comfortable: the breasts usually become engorged when the milk first comes in (about four days after the birth) and leaking is common. But repeated studies show that only a small percentage of postpartum women who don't nurse experience serious pain from breast engorgement. Breast engorgement is a temporary and medically benign condition that can generally be treated with over-the-counter pain medications, cold compresses, and tight chest wrappings. The FDA studied women who chose to forgo medication and found that well over 90% required no pain medication, with the most painful period lasting approximately twelve hours. Additionally, there are no health hazards involved in letting nature take its course. This is not the case with lactation-suppressing drugs.

Lactation-suppressing drugs can be hormones, such as estrogens, or medicines that shift the body chemistry. Doctors have routinely prescribed lactation suppressants despite the fact that only a small percentage of women ask for them. The drugs have well-documented side effects. Nausea, dizziness, headaches, vomiting, abdominal cramps, diarrhea, and lightheadedness are among the mild symptoms. Heart attacks, strokes, seizures, blood clots in the lungs, and severe high or low blood pressure are among the serious side effects reported. Most of the recipients of these drugs are not informed about the side effects, nor are they told that they could have potentially life-threatening reactions.

Since 1989, the only drug specifically approved for lactation suppression has been bromocriptine mesylate, marketed under the brand name Parlodel. Sold by Sandoz Pharmaceuticals, Parlodel stops the pituitary gland in the brain from secreting prolactin, the hormone that stimulates milk production. A two-week supply of the drug costs about $40. Critics say that Parlodel has been responsible for hundreds of serious side effects in new mothers, including dozens of seizures, strokes, and heart attacks in the past decade—at least thirteen of them fatal.

The FDA has been well aware of these risks. As far back as 1983, reports were clear that the risks of these drugs outweighed the benefits. In 1989, the FDA asked the pharmaceutical companies for a voluntary cessation of the drugs; at that time all lactation suppressants except Parlodel were taken off the market. In September 1993, Public Citizen Health Research Group urged the FDA to order Parlodel off the market for lactation suppression (the drug is also approved for treating the symptoms of Parkinson's disease and various endocrine disorders, for which its safety is not being challenged). The company responded with statements that the drug has been prescribed to more than seven million new mothers since it was approved for use in 1980, and that pregnancy-related hormonal changes naturally leave some women at increased risk of a stroke or heart attack in the first weeks after delivery (so that the medical problems blamed on the drug might well have happened anyway).

Seven weeks after the Public Citizen warning, Robin Snow, a twenty-two-year-old Texan, gave birth to a daughter and decided not to breastfeed. Her doctor prescribed Parlodel to dry up her milk. Six days later, she suffered a heart attack and seizures that left her paralyzed and semicomatose. Her parents filed suit against Sandoz Pharmaceuticals, her doctors, and the hospital. This was only the latest in a series of lawsuits against Sandoz for Parlodel. In July 1994, the first case was settled. A jury in Kentucky ordered Sandoz to pay $2 million to a thirty-six-year-old mother who is partially paralyzed from a stroke she suffered while taking Parlodel after a pregnancy in 1988 (Sandoz has appealed the verdict).

In August 1994, Public Citizen continued its attacks against Parlodel by filing a lawsuit against the FDA to force the agency to restrict the medication's use. After the suit was filed, the FDA announced that it would formally withdraw its approval for Parlodel for postpartum breast engorgement. Twenty-four hours later, Sandoz announced it was "voluntarily" changing its labeling of the drug to omit its use for lactation suppression.

The matter has not ended, however. Doctors can still legally prescribe Parlodel to new mothers (doctors may prescribe any drug that is sold legally; since Parlodel is still sold for other medical conditions, there is no bar against its use for lactation suppression). This fear may be well grounded if Sandoz convinces doctors that it changed its position as a response to political and legal pressures, not as a result of safety concerns. Even though Parlodel sales in the United States account for less than $25 million of Sandoz's $10.3 billion annual worldwide sales, the company is not anxious to lose a market that it dominates.

The tragedy of lactation-suppression drugs is that doctors have aggressively directed their patients to take ineffective, dangerous substances from which the drug makers have profited handsomely and which have the FDA's blessing—all in an effort to enable women to free themselves from the "burden" of providing their newborn with the most superior food available. These medicines are going to women who know little about breastfeeding and who have expressed an unwillingness even to try it! It would be easy to blame the women for being so selfish that they would endanger their health rather than let their own child suckle from their breast. But the FDA, the medical profession, and the drug makers are the real culprits. What kind of society have we created that will direct so many resources at stopping lactation—and so few at encouraging it?

ADDING UP THE PIECES

There is an illusory complacency about the effects of bottle-feeding. America today has the sad distinction of having the lowest breastfeeding rate of all industrialized nations. Many people prefer to believe that there is no relationship between these two statistics.

During the period following World War II, bottle-feeding became the "normal" method of baby feeding in the United States and to a lesser extent in Europe (Figure 3.8). The breastfeeding rate fell by half between 1946 and 1956, and by 1967 only 25% of American babies were being breastfed at the time of hospital discharge. In comparison, in Australia and throughout Scandinavia, breastfeeding at the time of hospital discharge is almost universal. Ironically, the only statistics available on breastfeeding in America are those collected and compiled by formula companies. Today in America, only 54% of new mothers are breastfeeding (not exclusively, however) when they take their newborns home. As few as one baby in five has *any* breastmilk at all when five months old. Even though breastfeeding rates are on the increase today, it is the more educated, more affluent women who account for the increase. Poor women, especially young poor women with the fewest resources and the greater proportion of at-risk babies, often don't even consider breastfeeding their children. Some of the blame for this goes to the government-sponsored WIC (Women, Infants, and Children) program, which is perceived as promoting formula-feeding.

In developing countries, breastfeeding rates, and especially exclusive breastfeeding, have declined markedly (Figure 3.9). Three trends have contributed to this: mixed feeding (combining bottle and breast), discarding colostrum and providing prelacteal feeds, and early introduction of solids. In addition to these trends there is a practice of "bottling the breast." This has caused a rise in infant mortality. To counteract this, a number of new breastfeeding promotion, support, and protection programs have been undertaken. Dr. Clavano, working in the Philippines, showed that, by introducing rooming-in and exclusive breastfeeding in the hospital, there was a decrease in infant mortality as well as decreases in neonatal sepsis, infantile diarrhea, and the use of intravenous fluids. From the hospital's point of view, this was extremely economical and reduced hospital costs. Breast-

Figure 3.8
Breastfeeding Rates in the United States

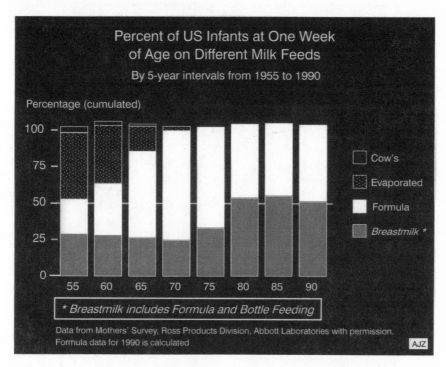

Percent of US Infants at One Week of Age on Different Milk Feeds
By 5-year intervals from 1955 to 1990

Percentage (cumulated)

* Breastmilk includes Formula and Bottle Feeding

Data from Mothers' Survey, Ross Products Division, Abbott Laboratories with permission.
Formula data for 1990 is calculated

feeding rates went up dramatically in a country where bottle-feeding was becoming the norm. This was then followed by other programs at the José Fabella Hospital in Quezon City, Philippines, where there was a significant decrease in the hospital's consumption of milk formula, bottles, nipples, water, and power for sterilization. Staff costs were also reduced. A savings of $107,297 was realized in 1989 alone. The space for the central nursery is now being used for rooming-in wards, but most importantly, there are no cases of neonatal diarrhea and sepsis.

In 1986, the major maternity hospital in Quito, Ecuador, a public hospital facilitating more than 14,000 births annually, committed itself to the promotion of breastfeeding. Although chronically understaffed, a decision was made to cease all use of infant formulas. Newborns would receive only their mother's milk; milk donated from mothers within the hospital would be used for those babies who needed supplementing. This one policy change alone led to a dramatic decline in neonatal infection and mortality rates.

Just because infant formula is the best alternative to breastmilk is not to say that the difference between a live biological fluid and a dead processed

Figure 3.8 (continued)

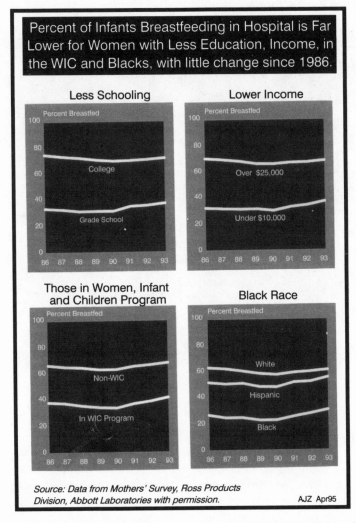

Note: The survey definition of breastfeeding was imprecise and included added bottle-feeding.

one is insignificant. No one who even remotely understands the miracle of breastmilk could possibly say that the choice between formula and breast-feeding is simply one of convenience. Formula makers insist that maternal convenience comes from having anyone be able to feed your baby; breast-feeding mothers tell you that the ultimate convenience is having your own self-contained, unlimited milk supply. As the debate goes on, formula companies ring up tremendous profits in what is now a $1.5 billion per year

Figure 3.9
Percentage of Infants 0–4 Months Exclusively Breastfed in Developing
Countries, by Country

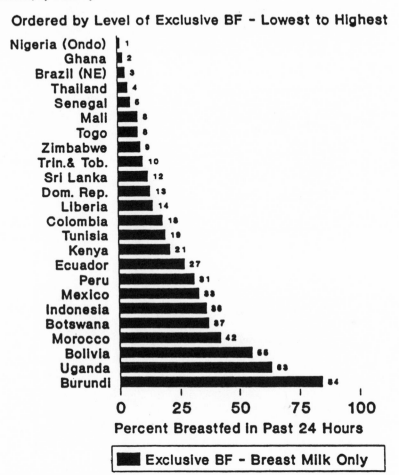

Source: USAID. Data from Demographic Health Surveys, 1986–89, Columbia,
Maryland.

business. Breastmilk is likely to be a source of continuing debate, with
advocates of all positions using arguments ranging from consumer choice
and corporate freedom to issues of employee entitlements and the health
of America's next generation.

Four

Artificial Feeding

The multitude of infant foods and substitutes for mother's milk suggests the conclusion that none are completely successful, and the startling mortality statistics would be conclusive evidence did any doubt exist. So long as the medical profession relegates its thinking to commercial men, the market will continue to be flooded with "baby foods" and the figures of infant mortality repeat themselves with sickening regularity.

—A.C. Cotton, *Care of Children*, 1907

INFANTS DIE LIKE FLIES

Until the nineteenth century, artificial feeding was a recipe for certain disaster. Although a wide variety of products and feeding methods were tried, failure remained the most frequent outcome. It was the exceptionally rare child who survived on hand- or dry-feeding, as artificial feeding was then called. Underwood, an eighteenth-century physician, estimated that only one in eight hand-fed infants in London survived, a fact he attributed to those babies' superior genes rather than to any specific food source.

Infant survival, even among those exclusively breastfed, was hardly something to be taken for granted. In the mid-1760s in London, there were an average of 16,283 births a year and an annual number of burials of children under age two of 7,987: almost half the children born in London were dead within two years, and another 26% died before they turned five. In the last century, infant mortality rates were as high as 400 per thousand babies born (in developed countries, the 1991 figure was 8 deaths per thousand live births; in developing countries, it ranged from 84 to 188 per 1000 live births). The major cause of death was diarrhea. (This is still the case. A 1985 study from an urban area in southern Brazil found that bottle-fed babies are fourteen times more likely to die from diarrhea than those exclusively breastfed.)

While we come from a perspective where heroic measures are often undertaken to save any baby, this was not always the situation. Generally speaking, last century's medicine men were not particularly focused on studying and/or saving infants. They typically held babies in low regard, viewed them as miniature adults, and often ignored their welfare. The lack of concern for children was largely due to issues of class. Though the rich could afford to hire wet nurses, their infant mortality was high; but infant mortality was even higher in the infants of the lower and middle classes whose infants were most at risk. These infants were considered a dime-a-dozen and of no particular importance.

It is interesting to look at the church's outlook. Instead of being concerned with the wastage of life as a vile human tragedy, church officials regarded it as a "suitable fate for the offspring of harlots since it prevented them from perpetuating the sins of their mothers." The Catholic church has since done an about-face and now advocates both limiting the access to birth control and employing costly and extensive measures to save each and every new life.

It was men outside of the medical and denominational leadership, like Thomas Coram, who, appalled by the stench of infants rotting on dung heaps, took it upon themselves to change the system. In the mid-eighteenth century, Coram exposed this deplorable situation and caused a public outcry which resulted in the establishment of the first foundling home in England. Unfortunately, in spite of the well-meaning intentions, conditions in these foundling homes were so appalling that it is surprising any infants survived. Of the 15,000 infants admitted to the foundling hospital, more than 10,000 died in infancy. In some London parishes around 1750, the mortality ranged from 80–90%, while that of those younger than one year of age was even higher (Rosen, 1958).

While in most parts of the world little was attempted, and even less was successful, there were some notable efforts to reduce the high rates of infant mortality. In the South of France, an outstanding effort was made in 1852 by Monsignor Morel, the mayor of Villiers-le-duc, who initiated a program to stem the wastage of life. He did this by offering a bounty to mothers whose breastfed infants lived to see their first birthday. By doing this, he succeeded in lowering the infant mortality rate by 33%.

In 1893, his son, who succeeded him as mayor, extended the maternity and child welfare program that his father had started. On reporting her pregnancy, every woman was visited by a physician who would then be responsible for both the mother's and infant's care during pregnancy and after birth. The infants were weighed biweekly and their progress charted. An intensive campaign was mounted to see that every mother nursed her baby for at least one year and to provide a wet nurse if she could not do

Figure 4.1
Infant Mortality in Nineteenth-Century Bavaria

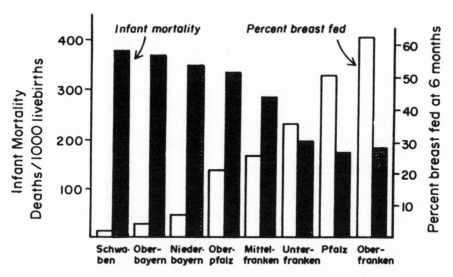

In Bavaria, in the late nineteenth century, there was a striking association between breastfeeding practices and infant mortality. The graph shows rates by district. *Source*: Data from J. Knodel and E. van der Walle, "Breast Feeding, Fertility and Infant Mortality," *Population Studies* 21, 1967.

so. In addition, the community maintained a herd of cows to supply clean milk to mothers and older children. The young Morel deduced that maintaining good health for the mothers was vital to successful breastfeeding and child rearing (a fact that has gone unnoticed by an astounding number of health professionals). By taking care of the children's nutrition, he also reduced their susceptibility to infection. Under this comprehensive program, the infant mortality at Villiers-le-duc dropped to zero over the ten-year period 1893–1903.

Contrast this to villages in nineteenth-century Bavaria, where breastfeeding was considered immoral and disgusting. The infant mortality was exceptionally high, and essentially all (96%) of the fatal cases of diarrhea came from the artificially fed infants (Figure 4.1). Unfortunately, the high infant mortality rate in the village didn't cause the townspeople to alter their attitude to breastfeeding.

In 1792, Jean Jacques Rousseau, the renowned French philosopher, had a great influence on how middle- and upper-class parents reared their children following the publication of his book *Emile*, in which he made his famous protest against the disinclination of French mothers to nurse their own children, citing it as a source of weakness to the nation. Unfortunately, just a few pages after this passage, in one of those inconsistencies which

Table 4.1
Mortality Rates in European Foundling Hospitals in the Eighteenth Century

Hospital	Dates	No. of Deaths (and % Mortality)	Feeding Method
London	1741–59	7,833 (56.0%)	wet nursing
Paris	1773–77	25,476 (80.0%)	wet nursing
Dublin	1775–96	10, 227 (99.6%)	dry nursing

Source: Short, Roger, "Breastfeeding, Fertility and Population Growth," ACC/SCN Symposium Report, Nutrition Policy Discussion Paper No. 11. ACC/SCN 18th Session Symposium, UNICEF, New York, August, 1993.

were so frequent in his life and works, Jean Jacques hired a wet nurse for
the infant Emile. He chose as a wet nurse a woman who had recently borne
a daughter and then proceeded to completely disregard her welfare. He
personally didn't practice what he preached—he sent his own five children
to a foundling hospital at birth, never to be seen by him again. In his later
years he made fruitless attempts to trace them.

In England, hired wet nurses experienced their heyday at the end of the
eighteenth century. Wet nurses usually received a significant sum of 25
guineas a year or, sometimes, ten a quarter, for their services. To meet the
job description, young unmarried women would deliberately conceive a
child. Sadly, the child was generally allowed to die a death of neglect
through "baby farming" or in foundling hospitals, as the new mothers
needed to be freed up for employment.

At that time, the infant mortality in Europe as well as England was
appalling (Table 4.1). Of 31,951 children admitted to the Paris Foundling
Hospital, for example, during 1773–77, fully 80% (25,476) died before
reaching their first birthday, compared to a death rate of 50% (7,601 out
of 15,104) during 1820–22, when public health had undergone some improvements. At the Dublin Foundling Asylum during 1775–96, where dry
nursing was in vogue, only 45 children survived out of 10,272—a horren-
dous 99.6% mortality rate.

By the end of the nineteenth century, the increase in the number of foundlings and the finding that a high mortality rate in infants was associated
with artificial feeding resulted in renewed efforts to find ways to improve
infant hygiene and to make better breastmilk substitutes available. Artificial
feeding brought with it many challenges. What was clearly needed was an
effective and uncontaminated container for feeding the infant and an effective and uncontaminated liquid to feed to the infant. The number of
areas where errors could be made in the feeding process or the product
were astronomical. For instance, cow's milk was often "dirty," typically

the rich butterfat was skimmed off and saved for the adults, and, routinely, the milk was further diluted with contaminated water. Even if cow's milk were, in and of itself, a viable alternative food for newborns, the substance actually fed to the newborns was a poor imitation of the real thing (Figure 4.2).

It was absolutely impossible for artificial feeding to become less lethal until several major milestones were achieved. First and foremost, the general state of public health had to be upgraded, by acts such as chlorination of water (which began in 1880), improved methods of sewage disposal, and stricter regulation of dairy herd housing and feeding (to protect raw milk from bacterial contamination). Safe methods of storing, transporting, and handling the milk also had to be developed. What initially appeared to be a simple problem to solve proved to be much more difficult than anyone had thought.

CLEAN MILK

Each public hygiene measure that contributed to the safety of artificial infant foods brought marked improvement to the community. For example, before these health measures were adopted, cows (which were commonly diseased with tuberculosis and skin infections) were housed in dirty, damp stables, were so sick that they had to be propped up to be milked (Figure 4.3), and were fed distillery mash or other discarded materials. These distillery cows produced "swill milk" which, among other things, succeeded in intoxicating the infants. While a tipsy child was perhaps a blessing for a babysitter, it wasn't good for the baby.

It was the French bacteriologist Louis Pasteur and his new-found ability to destroy germs through gentle heating who did away with these milk-borne infections. Pasteur, who revolutionized ideas about the origin of disease, was the first to show that living things came only from other living things and disproved the then-current notion of spontaneous generation. It was thought that fermentation occurred spontaneously, the way maggots were thought to arise spontaneously from putrefied meat. In 1857, Pasteur determined that the process of fermentation was actually brought about by feeding yeast organisms. He concluded that spoilage of perishable products could be prevented by destroying the microbes present and protecting the sterilized material against future contamination. Pasteur found that gently heating liquids destroyed most of the microbes without significantly altering the flavor. (By developing this heating process, Pasteur also saved the wine industry from collapse.) His name became a household word: to pasteurize is to use heat to partially sterilize liquids. Today, almost all fresh milk, wine, and beer sold in the United States is pasteurized.

Additionally, as public health became more of a concern, a "clean milk"

Figure 4.2
Impure Milk as a Cause of Infant Death

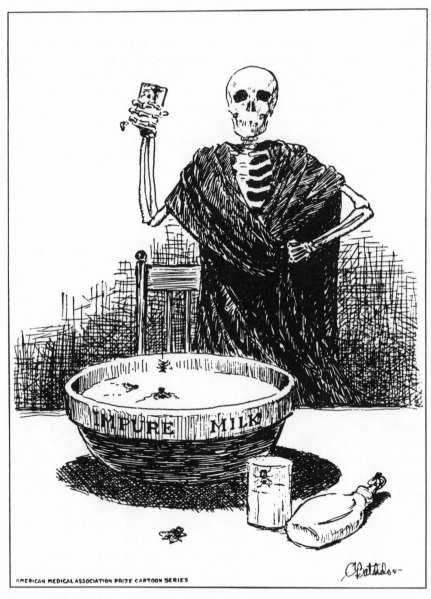

AMERICAN MEDICAL ASSOCIATION PRIZE CARTOON SERIES

Source: Lina Strauss, *Diseases in Milk*. 2nd ed. (New York: Dutton, 1917). *Photo courtesy*: History of Medicine Division, National Library of Medicine, Bethesda, Maryland.

Figure 4.3
Impure Milk

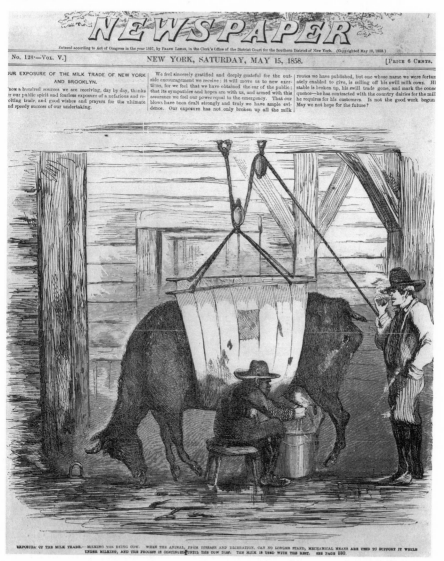

A diseased cow, unable to stand, is hoisted up in order to be milked. *Source: Harper's Weekly*, May 15, 1858.

movement was started. The milkers themselves were instructed to practice hygiene and were required to use veterinarians to screen the animals for diseases such as typhoid and tuberculosis (some outbreaks of these diseases were linked to milkers who did not know they were carriers of the disease).

This clean milk movement was very important, as it mandated stricter control and quality assurance of milk. Sterilization by boiling became an established practice. Milk certification was started and meant that consumers could rely on some measure of product control. Of course, these improvements did not come without cost. The price of certified milk was double the cost of regular milk, and even though the milk was much safer, it still could cause health problems such as tuberculosis.

Physicians began to demonstrate through studies that infants survived if they were given boiled milk. Despite this finding, many physicians, such as Dr. Coit in New York, firmly held that sterilization and pasteurization were harmful. Coit advocated "certified" milk, that is, clean but unpasteurized milk. But the certified milk theory was discredited when a herd of "certified cows" was found to be riddled with tuberculosis.

Cost was not the only thing that changed as a result of the certification process. The taste of pasteurized milk was different from raw milk, and advocates of raw milk believed that only raw milk contained the necessary "essential vital elements." To compound matters, some physicians in the late eighteenth and early nineteenth centuries recommended their patients give preference to "raw milk" and bypass the pasteurized variety. (Some people still believe that some of milk's vitality is destroyed by heating and prefer to drink only "raw milk," which can be purchased in health food stores.)

Another problem was that milk often soured while being transported. A hundred years ago, refrigeration was primitive, and even though the milk was pasteurized, the journey from farm to kitchen left many a bottle of spoilt milk. Milk fed to infants was particularly lethal in the summer months, when diarrhea was a major cause of death among bottle-fed infants. The widespread use of factory and household refrigeration has made many people forget what a risky product milk was until relatively recently, even in industrialized countries. Outbreaks of epidemics of diarrheal disease in 1929 and 1936 were milk borne. Indeed, the development and widespread use of the icebox played a major role in extending the safety and shelf life of milk.

Milk had long been used as a beverage for children, but its use for infants was relatively new. As more knowledge of the composition of breastmilk accumulated, cow's milk was modified or "humanized" and treated in a variety of ways to reduce the tough curds and make it more digestible. The method most commonly used was to dilute it with water and add sugar or barley water. The first proprietary formula was developed by a German chemist, Liebig, in 1867. He called his formula the "perfect food" for infants. It was made of cow's milk, flour, potassium bicarbonate, and malt. Although it was patented and commercialized and delivered in liquid form, it did not sell very well. Then a powder was developed and some of the cow's milk was replaced by pea flour, but it too appears to have received a poor reception. Liebig was quite annoyed by doctors who reported his food was indigestible or who doubted that it was the counterpart of mother's milk. Liebig is also credited with introducing condensed milk for infant feeding.

Introducing the public to different milks soon became a major business (Figure 4.4). Condensed milk was first developed and patented by Newton in 1835. It was made by boiling milk and then evaporating it to one-fourth of its original volume, with significant amounts of sugar (six ounces per pint) added as a preservative. At first it was sold in wax-capped bottles until 1866, when Nestlé marketed the first condensed milk in tin boxes. It was soon observed that prolonged feeding of infants on condensed milk gave rise to rickets (Vitamin D deficiency) and scurvy (Vitamin C deficiency), and several pediatric texts written at that time warned of these complications. Borden was one of the main producers of condensed milk. Anglo-Swiss, which later became Nestlé, was also an important supplier of condensed milk. By 1911, no fewer than one hundred varieties of machine-skimmed and forty brands of full-cream condensed milk had been marketed. Milks that did not require refrigeration provided a major breakthrough. The introduction of condensed and evaporated milks (evaporated milk was developed in 1885) meant that for the first time in history a baby could be fed cow's milk without the family having access to a cow.

Condensed milk had several distinct advantages over fresh milk. It was safe (as the milk had been boiled) and it was easy to store (as it required no refrigeration). Its acceptance was buoyed by extensive advertising. Free gifts were offered: baby diaries, book samples, fans, even chef-cooked meals for those who visited the factory.

In Paris, Pierre Budin, a well-known obstetrician concerned with high infant mortality, believed that providing sterilized milk at low cost to mothers, ready-bottled for each infant feed, was the answer. He started infant milk stations where infants were weighed weekly and their progress charted. If the infants did not gain satisfactorily, bottled sterilized milk was prescribed. This milk could be obtained from the milk stations or "Gouttes de Lait," as they were called.

As the practice developed of mothers coming regularly to the milk stations, the routine of weighing infants took hold. The custom of weighing infants, something every mother today assumes is part of her postpartum life, was only introduced a century ago. This "scientific" craze of weighing in and comparing the result to a weight chart caught on like wildfire. For the first time, there was an external, objective way of measuring whether

Figure 4.4
Early Promotion of Formula—Images and Messages

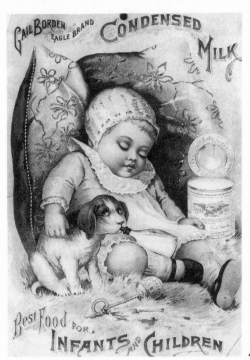
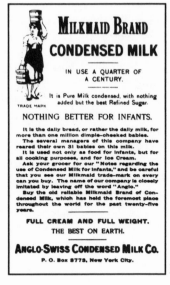

A   B

Trading cards that had enticing pictures on one side and product information on the other were used for advertising - (A) This advertisement for Eagle Brand Condensed Milk used a picture of a rich bonny contented baby girl with a caption "best food for infants"; (B) An example of an advertisement of Anglo-Swiss Condensed Milk Co. on the back of one of these trading cards. *Photo courtesy*: Warshaw Collection of Business Americana, Archives Center, National Museum of American History, neg. no. 357.

a child was thriving. This phenomenon took hold so much so that, in 1913, a physician named Cran commented in the British medical journal *Lancet* that the weighing machine had become an instrument of torture as much to the mother with plenty of milk as to the mother whose lactation was poor.

   Milk stations were soon all the fashion (Figure 4.5). At the turn of the century, "milk depots" were established in France, Britain, and the United States with the declared aim of providing uncontaminated milk for babies. In New York, Nathan Strauss of Macy's, working through health department clinics, organized milk stations where pasteurized, bottled milk was provided free for the needy and at low cost to others. These milk stations later evolved into well-child care clinics. The primary object of the clinics was to encourage mothers to breastfeed and, when breastfeeding was not possible, to provide safe and effective substitution. Special bottled formula and teats were supplied to mothers with infants. Different formulas were prepared and prescribed for three age groups of infants. Mothers were instructed in the proper feeding and care of children. It was said that the milk stations saved the lives of many infants.

EDUCATION AND ADVERTISING

While there is no question that the milk stations played a significant role, other measures also played a part. Health education, pioneered in New York's lower East Side, included home visits to the homes of all registered newborns by public health visitors and/or nurses. Dr. Josephine Baker, a public health doctor in New York, was able to show in the summer of 1908 that this type of preventive program resulted in a considerable reduction in infant mortality.

Dr. Baker understood that good hygienic practices were necessary and good mothering was essential. She started "the little mother leagues" among school girls and gave them practical instruction in child care. The girls served as missionaries of the new gospel in the tenements and slums. Dr. Baker knew that when the mother worked, the little girl in the family was "the little mother" and as such was a good target of an educational campaign.

In England, the milk stations, or rather the "child welfare clinics," provided powdered milk marketed as Glaxo, which was imported from New Zealand. This was sold at the child welfare clinics for half the store price. The Truby King program, operating in New Zealand, was also implemented in England: nurses were trained to visit mothers with newborns in their homes and talk to them about the child's well-being. If the infants were not gaining weight and the mother was suspected of having little milk, milk samples were collected and tested for fat content.

Truby King, whose ideas came largely from veterinary science, helped to successfully reestablish breastfeeding. His main flaw was an obsession with the clock. While he called it Truby King's "natural way," mothers were instructed to feed on a regimented schedule instead of by demand. In a 1925 report on infant feeding there was the regretful statement that "some mothers had not even seen a clock and those who had, could not understand what it had to do with the feeding of an infant."

The obsession with regimented feeding was the result of anxiety about severe diarrhea. Known as "the summer complaint," severe diarrhea afflicted thousands of babies each summer. The causes of this potentially life-

Figure 4.5
Distribution of Milk

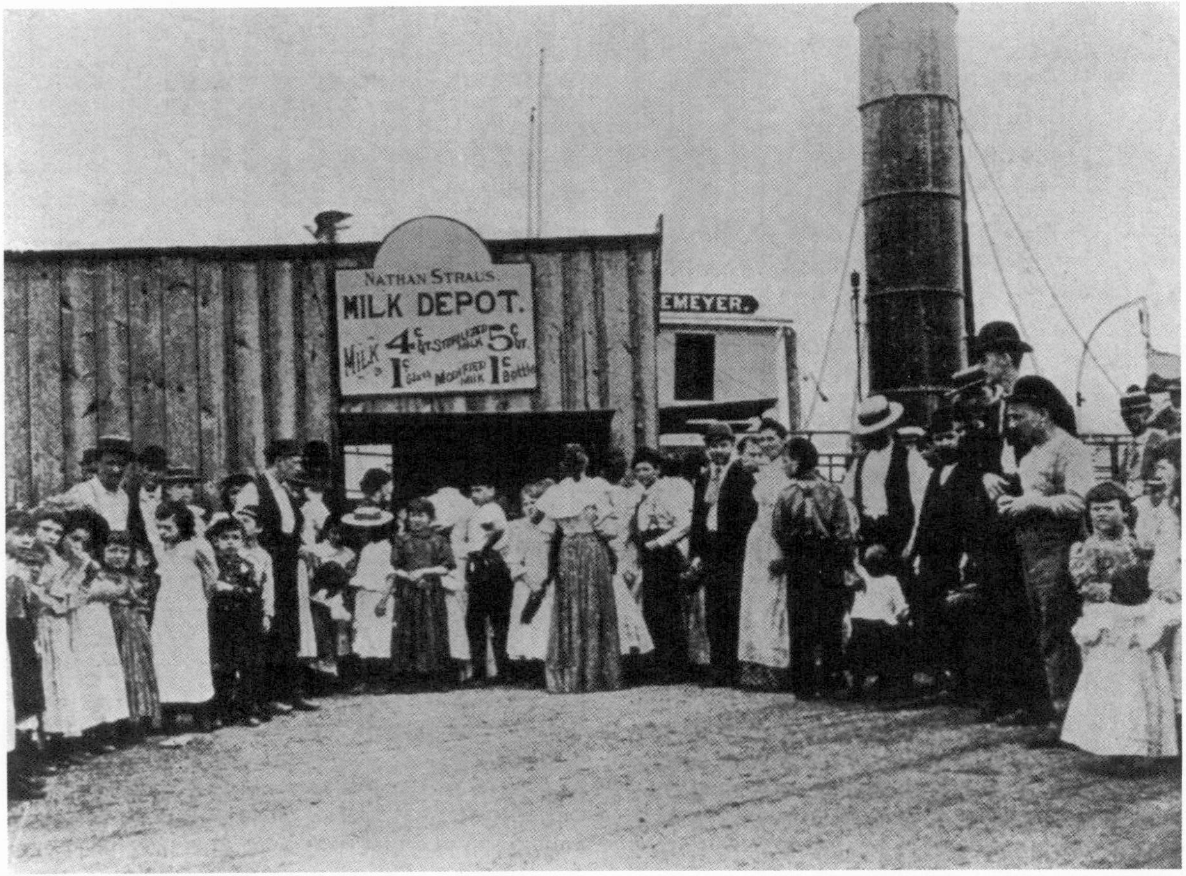

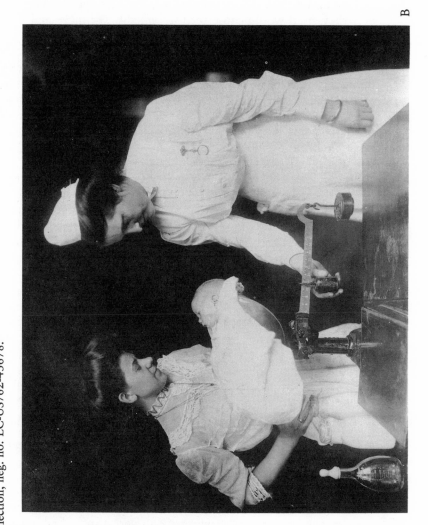

(A) A milk station in New York earlier in this century. *Source:* Lina Strauss, *The Diseases of Milk.* 2d ed. (New York: Dutton, 1917). *Photo courtesy:* History of Medicine Division, National Library of Medicine, Bethesda, Maryland. (B) A weighing station in a Cincinnati health clinic. These centers became milk stations and, if the infant was not gaining enough, bottle-feeding was advised. *Photo courtesy:* Library of Congress Photo and Prints Division, Bain Collection, neg. no. LC-US762-43678.

B

threatening disease were believed to include irregular feeding schedules. Doctors put the fear of God into mothers, persuading them to ignore the hungry pleas of their children until the next scheduled feed.

It wasn't until the early 1940s that bacterial contamination and inadequate refrigeration were found to be the culprits of the summer complaint. During all this time, the common wisdom held that feeding babies whenever they cried would cause them to greedily cry more and more often. A simple but bold experiment conducted in the early 1940s by Frances Simsarian, a new mother and psychologist, and her pediatrician, Preston McLendon, changed the conventional thought on scheduled feedings. They decided to see what would happen if Frances allowed her newborn to nurse at the breast whenever the baby seemed hungry. Within a few days, the baby settled into a schedule of feeding six or seven times a day. The effect of this experiment on pediatric medicine was dramatic and profound—in a very short time, doctors went from advising rigid feeding schedules to advocating extreme flexibility.

But back to Truby King. While he was educating mothers in the virtues of clock-watching, he also made efforts to ensure the mothers were also educated about artificial feeding methods in case their breastmilk was insufficient. This preparation for failure may have contributed to lactation failure, as it has been repeatedly shown that the availability and promotion of alternative foods usually has a demoralizing effect on both individual and social confidence in breastfeeding.

According to Ebrahim, a professor at the Institute of Child Health in London, as the number of milk child welfare clinics increased so did the sale of Glaxo's powdered milk. Milk stations really took off and became a fashionable solution to infant mortality. In 1903, at an international meeting on the Gouttes de Lait, which took place in Paris, the obstetricians attending the meeting accused the pediatricians of making mothers stop breastfeeding by recommending artificial milk through the milk stations.

One of the largest producers of condensed milk was Gail Borden's company called the New York Condensed Milk Company. At least one member of the Borden family was involved in the public health department's milk stations that Dr. Josephine Baker had started. Condensed milk was well advertised and a big seller at this time. As part of their advertising campaign, Anglo-Swiss produced picture cards that stated how big their operation was even then:

Six factories in operation, employing 700 workingmen condensing the milk of 13,000 cows and producing 20 millions of 1 pound cans per year an amount equal to 1,000 car loads, or to a loaded train 5 miles in length, and a sufficient number of cans, if placed side by side in a single land, to make a row of milk cans over 1,000 miles long.

As further testimony, the advertisement continued:

This brand is sold by over 4,000 grocers in London alone and is becoming favorably known in America.

The American Condensed Milk Company, with offices in New York, was catering to the infant market as early as 1865. In one of their advertisements, a direct appeal to the mothers, the company boasted:

Safest milk for infants and children. . . . The names of many of our physicians and first class hotel keepers who are using this milk will be given for reference if desired. Ladies are respectfully invited to call at the office and judge the merits of the product themselves.

Nestlé, like other companies, also made high claims for its products, labeling its product in its advertisements as "indispensable as a diet for infants" and quoting a list of doctors as references. They also cited "Strumpels text" as the authority (whoever that might have been) and appealed to "scientific" minds and perhaps simply the fashionable. (This strategy of using medical doctors for testimonials is still being used today by the formula companies.) By 1873, Nestlé was selling 500,000 boxes of "farine lactée" per year in Europe, the United States, Argentina, Mexico, and the Dutch East Indies.

THE GROWTH OF ARTIFICIAL FOODS

The formulations for artificial baby milk are changed frequently and represent one of the largest uncontrolled experiments in altered nutrition for humankind ever conducted. (Kathleen Auerbach, *Journal of Tropical Pediatrics*, 1992)

The greatest need for breastmilk substitutes (BMS) was for the growing number of foundlings, sick babies, and nursery infants. Milk laboratories grew out of this need and started preparing doctor-tailored milk for infants. Barley, oats, lime juice, and sugar were among the commonest breastmilk supplements. Special ready-to-feed prescriptions were also created and made available for home delivery.

Initially, when these preparations came on the market, there was a significant amount of collusion between the manufacturers and the doctors (Figure 4.6). Several manufacturers were owned by doctors and pharmacists. They wanted doctors to sanction their products, while doctors wanted to retain control over the distribution of formula and share in the profits from this new market. Of course, this was not portrayed as collusion. Rather, it represented a great partnership of learned men demonstrating their commitment to infant nutrition. It was seen as "men of sense," rather than "foolish unlearned women," taking over the supervision of infant

Figure 4.6
Scientists and Doctors Endorse Products

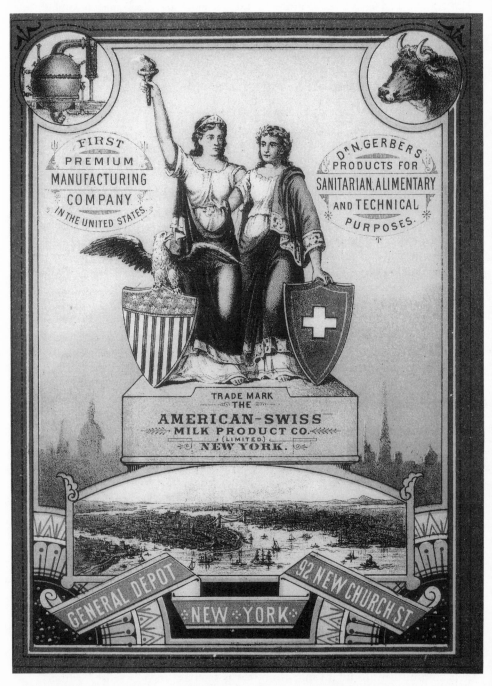

Advertisements from early on used doctors' names and quoted doctors as part of the sales pitch. *Photo courtesy*: Warshaw Collection of Business Americana, National Museum of American History.

care. In an affront to the notion of medical integrity, these endorsements were designed to relieve patients of their money rather than their suffering.

At first, physicians were involved by making up an individual "formula" to suit each child's particular digestion. Custom-made formulas were produced in the doctors' offices, supposedly crafted to meet the specific nutritional needs of each individual child (of course, it was only the rich who could afford this service). Obviously, optimal infant nutrition was not achieved, but there were a few beneficial effects from this degree of involvement by the medical profession. First, it promoted better hygiene. Second, doctors had more responsibility and involvement in the care of infants. When an infant failed to thrive or died while using a doctor's controlled formula, he was held accountable.

Custom-made formulas turned out to be impractical and, as the number of infants put on formula increased, individualizing prescriptions became too inconvenient and costly. In addition, excluding lower- and middle-class families, who could not afford private physician care, meant a large market was being ignored. The next step was mass production and widespread distribution of these proprietary products—but with no directions on the package. The instructions simply advised consumers to consult their doctors before using the product. Commercial baby foods were acknowledged to be dangerous when used without instruction, yet neither doctors nor manufacturers attempted to restrict or control their distribution. This was considered "ethical" marketing. Mead Johnson boasted with all honestly in 1923 that their "ethical" marketing policy was "responsible in large measure for the advancement of the profession of pediatrics in this country because it brought control of infant feeding under the direction of the medical profession."

Technological developments greatly added to the availability of formula ingredients. The mechanization of the dairy industries resulted in large surpluses of whey from the cheese industry, which in turn led to a major expansion of the baby milk industry during the late nineteenth and early twentieth centuries. Dried milk powder, produced through roller and spray drying, added to the availability of inexpensive and transportable milk. Buckets of skimmed milk were abundant as butter factories sought a profitable market for its waste.

Other preparations of altered milk also were developed and marketed for the young. Modifications to cow's milk were numerous. Curd size reduction was accomplished through acidification using such acids as tartaric, lactic, citric, or even acidified whey. Milk was also peptonized, or predigested, by pancreatin bicarbonate of soda and then added to milk powder. Such milk preparations were sold as "humanized milk." Allenbury's Peptonized Powder was one of many such preparations. Smith, Kline, and French produced a milk modifier called Eskays that "albuminized food." Eskays was complete with special instructions for each age group detailed in a free booklet, "How to care for the baby." The booklet listed stories of infants who were saved and subsequently thrived on the product. In the United States, Mellin's Milk Modifier was another of the creations marketed for infant feeding.

By the turn of the century, artificial foods were widely available, widely used, and widely advertised as the ultimate infant food, requiring only the addition of water (which also carried with it a fair share of health problems). As we know, there is a long journey from researchers' theories to the babies' stomachs and that the possibility of error is endless. Problems at the various levels—farm, factory, laboratory, packaging, transport, storage, and kitchen—can easily occur. Bacterial contamination was one such problem. An analysis of a batch of diluted Nestlé condensed milk, incubated at 98.6°F, for example, contained 11 million bacteria after twenty-four hours. But even if the formula manufactured was the perfect food source, safe hygiene was impossible in the average, overcrowded, ill-equipped home.

It wasn't long before problems were identified by consumers of these new milks. Cases of rickets (a bone disease resulting from a deficiency of Vitamin D) and scurvy (a Vitamin C deficiency) were linked to their consumption. It took some time to realize that when milk was boiled, there was a loss of a B vitamin called pyridoxine. Many of the infants fed only condensed milk or boiled milk developed convulsions and even beri beri. Problems also arose when dried skimmed milk was used, as it was Vitamin A deficient. As expected, the nutritional problems were not discovered until some time after the product had been on the market. In an effort to reduce the incidence of infantile malnutrition in Indonesia, relief agencies handed out dried milk powder that had not been fortified with Vitamin A. The result was untold misery, including a large number of children who developed Vitamin A deficiency blindness (xerophthalmia).

These products were marketed as new, modern, and exciting; they were presented as allowing women to reap the benefits of technological breakthroughs, providing mothers with more freedom and convenience than had ever been possible. Yet it was not uncommon for these artificial foods to lead to infant infection, malnutrition, anemia, brain damage, and death.

Not everyone jumped on the artificial foods bandwagon. Lionel Chalmers, a leading physician at the time, aptly stated: "Sensible parents will be content to leave the recipe [for infant formula] for some coming race who may prefer art to nature."

Unfortunately, Chalmers's advice was not widely heeded. By 1873, no fewer than twenty-seven brands of patented infant formula had appeared on the market. Each brand stated its superiority by implication and used testimonials to stress its excellence. Paying homage to the scientific theme, in 1911 a new formula was produced under the name of "Scientific Milk Adaptation" (SMA), in which cow's milk fat was replaced with a mixture of cod liver oil and beef tallow (an inexpensive waste product from the meat industry). One of the scientific objectives was to provide a fat iodine content equivalent to breastmilk iodine. But the fat was not only poorly absorbed, it also bound calcium and phosphorus and was potentially rickets producing. It took another twenty-five years for the milk to be appropriately changed.

One of the most distressing aspects of the growth of the artificial food industry is that ingredients have often been chosen more for their profitability than for their superior nutritional content. The most common fat used in formula is coconut oil because of its low cost and widespread availability. Beef tallow is also used for the same reason. Breastmilk substitutes are also made from soy beans, used mainly for infants with known or suspected allergies to cow's milk. This is not because a range of foods were analyzed to determine what sources of protein could be used to manufacture the best nondairy food source for babies, but rather, a vast and profitable soy bean industry aggressively sought out new outlets for its products.

Nowadays, formulas produced for infants use a mixture of vegetable oils such as coconut, cottonseed, and soya to replace the cow's milk fat (some still use beef tallow). The protein content too has been adjusted. Excess cheese whey has been used by baby formula manufacturers to make the cow's milk protein more digestible. Excess electrolytes are dialyzed off the whey and to this are added fat sugar and stabilizers, such as carageenan, to produce a variety of so-called "human" milks. It must be apparent by now that these concocted "human" milks are merely cow's milk, treated, altered, and added to in a vain attempt to replace the inimitable human milk. Today, baby milk is an $8 billion per year business!

FEEDING VESSELS

As stated before, not only was inventing a suitable artificial food a major challenge, but also developing a suitable means of holding and delivering the artificial food was almost as great a challenge. The biggest obstacle to the success of artificial feeding was not only creating an appropriate breastmilk substitute but also finding appropriate containers and imitation nipples. A full-term newborn usually has an excellent sucking reflex. For the infant to receive optimal nourishment, a feeding vessel must take advantage of this sucking reflex. The feeding contraptions devised over time look humorous now, but the large variety of types and styles invented indicates that each had its own problems and all are obsolete now. Figure 4.7 shows a sampling of feeding vessels.

Deterrents to most of these human-made devices included containers that were bacterial traps, instruments that either fed the child too quickly or too slowly, and objects that were cumbersome for the adult to handle. The

Figure 4.7
Types of Feeding Vessels

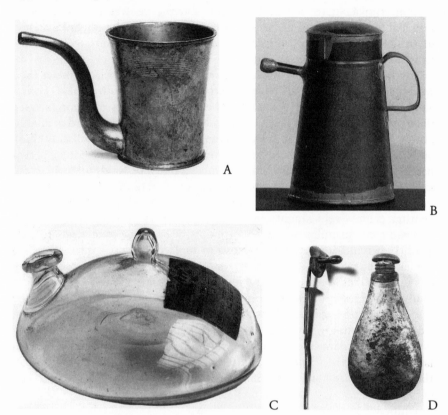

(A) Bubby-pot feeder developed by Hugh Smith in 1777. *Photo courtesy*: Wellcome Centre, Medical Photographic Library; (B) Pennsylvania Dutch tin nursing can. *Photo courtesy*: Cleveland Medical Library Association; (C) Infant nursing bottle, patented office model, 1868. Infant nursing bottle, lacteal patented in the United States in 1841. *Photo courtesy*: National Museum of American History, Medical and Science Collection, Smithsonian Institution, neg. no. 43090B; (D) Tin nursing bottle 1880s and silver nursing tube 1850s. *Photo courtesy*: National Museum of American History, Medical and Science Collection, Smithsonian Institution, neg. no. 43090A.

problem that most intrigued inventors of the nursing bottle was how to deal with the partial vacuum created when the infant fed. The physics of replacing the even flow of breastmilk by an artificial device was a dilemma that was irrespective of the shape of the container. It was not until the development of effective and inexpensive glass bottles and rubber nipples that infant formula became more attractive to consumers. It was the "pocket wet nurse," as the bottle/nipple became known, that revolutionized artificial feeding.

From available archeological finds, evidence exists that the search for an artificial feeding method is not new. Numerous civilizations have attempted to artificially duplicate a mother's breast. Infant nursing vessels were known to be used in Ancient Egypt; in the Nile basin (500 BC), objects identified as feeding containers have been uncovered in graves. These include a cup with a long spout, unearthed in the grave of three-month-old twins. The ancient Greeks used low and globular feeding bottles, while the vessels of the Romans resembled the modern jug and pot. The earliest known feeding bottles for administering animal milks to human infants date from about 4000 BC. Large numbers of these feeding vessels of different designs have been found in children's graves in Greece and Italy. Later instruments for feeding were even made out of clay (Figure 4.8).

Cow horns were used as feeders in the middle ages, and this practice was continued into the eighteenth century. The milk was sucked by the infant through a stitched parchment teat shaped like the finger of a glove. As with most of these primitive devices, they were hard to clean and acted as culture media for bacteria. This mode of feeding was associated with a high incidence of diarrheal disease that was often lethal.

In the eighteenth century, feeding devices known as "ceramic boats" were also in use. One version of this type of feeder was invented by an English physician named Hugh Smith, who in 1770 developed a pewter milk or "bubby-pot" feeder, the object of which was to imitate nature in making the infant labor for its food. His invention was an important stage in the evolution of the modern nursing bottle. In the United States in Pennsylvania, German parents created a modified version of the "bubby-pot" out of tin, calling it "mammale" ("little breast" or "little mother"). It was even possible to strap this contrivance to the breast to achieve "a more natural effect."

If the infant was still hungry after being offered milk, or when the infant's first tooth appeared, pap and panada were offered frequently as supplementary feeds. The use of pap and panada was one of the most ancient prescriptions in infant feeding. Pap was made from flour or bread cooked in water with or without milk. Panada was the term used for preparations of flour, cereal, or bread and butter that were combined with and cooked in a soup. According to Lionel Chalmers, "the preposterous manner of feeding infants with pap, and such indigestible foods nauseously sweetened, is highly censurable at all times." While he condemned the use of pap, he continued the harmful age old practice of prescribing daily sips of sweet wine diluted in water for infants. Pap and panada were often fed from special spoons or "boats." A pap boat was a vessel made from pewter, silver, or pottery that had a long spout. These often were difficult to clean and were a source of disease.

An extraordinary and dangerous technique employed in the quest for a

Figure 4.8
Early Feeding Bottle

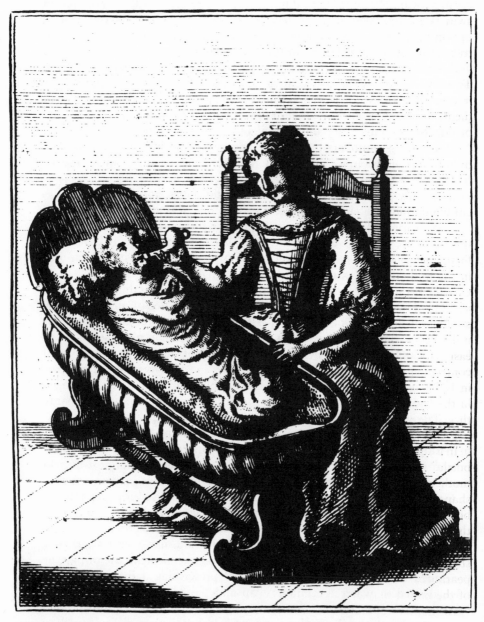

A woman feeding a baby in a crib using a clay bottle. *Source*: engraved frontis in *F. Baldini Metodo di Allatare a Mono i Bambini Napoli*, 1784. *Photo courtesy*: History of Medicine Division, National Library of Medicine, Bethesda, Maryland.

cheap artificial feeding method was the "sucking bag." This bag, popularized in Germany, was a by-product of the industrial age, replete with the crushing economic burden on family life and the employment of women in sweatshops, mines, and other industries. Working mothers had no other option but to devise some way to feed an infant while keeping their hands free for manual labor. Poor women made bags out of old shirts, filled them with bread, milk, and sugar, and popped one end into the infant's mouth. To make a bad situation worse, when the feeding bag fell onto the floor, it was picked up and pushed in the mouth again and again. This instrument, designed to nourish and console the infant, became a lethal source of infection.

Through the ages, many more feeding devices were fabricated, limited only by the imagination of the inventor. These included vessels fashioned out of wood, pewter, and even hog's stomachs. Some of these devices were prohibitively expensive and only available to the affluent. Most were patently lethal and summarily discarded.

It was the availability of glass as a construction material, combined with the technology for its mass production, that made the "pocket wet nurse" finally affordable to the lower classes. Glass feeding devices began to appear in the middle of the nineteenth century (Figure 4.9). In the United States, Charles Winship received the patent for the first infant glass feeding bottle in 1841. He called it a "patented lacteal." It was designed in the shape of a woman's breast, and, according to Winship, it induced "the child to think it derives nourishment from the mother." Apparently the children were not easily fooled, for the lacteal was quickly replaced by other devices. One contrivance that became quite popular was the O'Donnel bottle patented in 1851, to which long sucking tubes were attached. The tube was patented in the United States in 1864 and remained popular to the end of the century. The rubber tubes were a potent source of infection and it took twenty-five years for them to be taken off the market.

In 1868, another bizarre infant nursing bottle called the "Libbey Nursing bottle" made its debut. This bottle came equipped with a halter so that the mother could simulate breastfeeding by strapping a pair of these breast-shaped glass bottles around her torso in some way or another. In 1897, a bottle was patented that could be suspended over the cot and thus allowed the baby to feed with no adult nearby. Another bottle, with the same goal of parental independence, was designed with short legs so that it could stand unaided on the baby's chest. In 1869 "the Mamma" made its appearance; it was advertised as resembling the form, pliancy, and warmth of the breast (Figure 4.10).

All manner of contraptions have been developed for infant feeding purposes. As the number of infants artificially fed increased, so did these devices. Ida Simmons, a public health nurse working in the rural slums of Singapore in 1938, found the number of infants being fed artificially was

Figure 4.9
Unhygienic Bottle

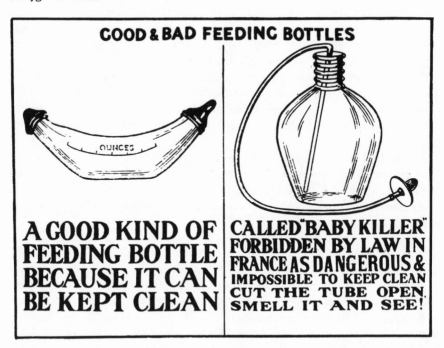

The use of glass bottles with long rubber tubing became fashionable in the 1880s. These bottles were recognized as a health hazard much later. This poster, designed by the Nurses Social Union of Kingston Grange Taunton, UK, in and around 1917, was used to warn mothers. *Source*: *Maternity and Child Welfare* 1, 167, 1917. *Photo courtesy*: Wellcome Centre Medical Photographic Library.

astonishingly high; they were kept in the dark, tightly bound, and in airless cubicles. One example she related showed how women's priorities and ingenuity could affect the infant's health adversely.

I once found ... a poor rickety baby sucking his milk from a large black bottle with a tube half a yard long connected to a thin hollow bamboo cane thrust through the hole of an empty cotton reel which formed the stopper. I gave the mother a hygienic feeder with a short teat and successfully fed the baby. For safety, I was proposing to take the tube outfit away. This caused great upset; the mother said "Oh yes, this is all right for the baby, but what will the pig do?" and disclosed a little suckling pig. ... The pig was being fattened for the Chinese New Year, the baby and pig were sharing one feeder.

A considerable amount of effort was spent in search of the perfect feeder, but the quest for a suitable nipple proved even more difficult. Duplicating

Figure 4.10
"The Mamma" Feeding Bottle

SAFE, CONVENIENT, AND HEALTHFUL NURTURE OF INFANTS.

MOST IMPORTANT INVENTION,
Specially approved by eminent Professional and Practical Authorities.

(ALL RIGHTS PROTECTED BY ROYAL LETTERS PATENT.)

J. PERRETT, SOLE PATENTEE.

"THE MAMMA"
INFANT'S (PATENT) FEEDING BOTTLE,

Which, from its unequalled properties of Simplicity, Convenience, and Comfort, is incomparably
superior to any substitute previously introduced, and must at once commend itself
to Mothers, and to all entrusted with the care of Infants.

ITS CONSTRUCTION — THE MOST SIMPLE.

ITS ACTION — THE NEAREST TO NATURE.

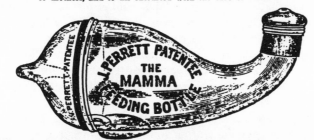

"THE MAMMA" INFANT'S (PATENT) FEEDING BOTTLE

Is the only one ever invented that supplies all the benefits derived from Nature itself, and thus overcomes the repugnance which sometimes renders it impossible to induce an Infant to take its food from a Bottle, in consequence of its missing the natural form, warmth, and pliant elasticity of the Breast.

The elastic part of this Bottle being moulded from Nature, the infant is at once attracted by it, and may be nursed with it from birth with the utmost ease; thus avoiding the difficulty and expense often experienced in obtaining a healthy and suitable wet-nurse.

Its perfect safety in use is one of its distinctive characteristics. In the first place, the danger of the Nipple coming off and choking the Infant—a mishap which has occurred not unfrequently—is avoided. Secondly, there being no tubes requiring brushes to cleanse them, the painful, irritating, and even fatal effects sometimes caused by bristles dropping from the brush into the tube, and passing thence into the Infant's throat, are likewise effectually precluded.

The Stopper of this Bottle is supplied with a valve identical in its action to the valve of the human heart, which enables the infant to take its food with the greatest ease, and at the same time (not allowing more air to enter the Bottle than is necessary) prevents the food from running out, no matter in what position the Bottle may be placed.

From the extremely simple construction of this unique Bottle, it can be kept constantly sweet and clean without the slightest trouble.

Ladies when nursing will, by cutting off the inner ring, find the Elastic Part form an admirable Shield.

Upon these grounds the Patentee respectfully submits that

"THE MAMMA" INFANT'S (PATENT) FEEDING BOTTLE

Possesses qualities wholly unapproached for efficacy in nurturing infants in a safe, convenient, comfortable, and salutary manner; and in this representation he is fortified, as already stated, by eminent and emphatically expressed opinions, which pronounce it an admirable and healthful substitute for Nature's Nursing.

DIRECTIONS FOR CLEANSING THE BOTTLE.—Remove the Elastic Band; take off the Breast; remove the Glass Tube and wash it out; turn the Breast inside out; wash it in either cold or warm water. The whole can be thoroughly cleansed in less than a minute.

*** *In cleansing this Bottle, it affords the peculiar advantage, over all others, of conveniently admitting the hand inside it.*

Price 3s. 6d. each.

SPARE BOTTLES, BREASTS, AND TUBES SUPPLIED SEPARATELY.

Sold by all Chemists and Druggists; and by J. PERRETT (Patentee),
at 35c, King-street, Cheapside, London, E.C.

BE CAREFUL TO SEE THAT THE NAME IS ON EACH BOTTLE AND BREAST.

This new invention was widely advertised as having the natural form, pliant elasticity, and warmth of the breast. *Source*: *Medical Times and Gazette*, 1869. *Photo courtesy*: History of Medicine Division, National Library of Medicine, Bethesda, Maryland.

the intricacies of a woman's anatomy was much more difficult than it appeared to be. Artificial nipples were tried in a variety of different forms and were fabricated out of an assortment of different materials. Sometimes the nipples were a part of the container when made of glass, pewter, wood, or even ivory. Other inventors made them a separate component, shaped out of parchment, chamois leather, linen, sponge, and even actual teats of cows soaked in spirits (alcoholic liquids were used to preserve and clean the devices). Unfortunately, unlike a real nipple, artificial nipples leaked and became infected.

The use of rubber as a material for fabricating teats was hardly an instant success. First patented in 1856, rubber teats were considered smelly, unyielding, and foul tasting. It was not until well into the twentieth century, after considerable modifications, that they became acceptable—and then only with aggressive advertising. Even though they are now the norm, as one eminent pediatrician declared, "The rubber teat is but a poor imitation of a mother's nipple." New ones now are even vanilla flavored.

The human nipple is pliable; it stretches 2–3 times its resting state, non-suckled length when in the infant's mouth. It contains 15–30 pores, each of which spurts milk in a fine stream in different directions. When the milk ejection reflex is activated, the spurts occur rhythmically throughout each nursing period.

The manufactured rubber teat and pacifier has a permanently erect shape, contains a single hole often so large that the stream of fluid through will cause choking if infant does not take defensive action by thrusting its tongue against the teat to stop the milk flow in order to swallow. The rubber may also be difficult to compress.

One notable device that was invented was fashioned to keep women's breasts hidden. This "anti-embarrassment device," patented in 1910, would supposedly allow women to breastfeed modestly in public (Figure 4.11). The inventor's description is worth noting:

The primary object of this invention is an improved construction or device for use by mothers with nursing infants, and designed particularly to avoid unpleasant and embarrassing situations in which mothers are sometimes placed in public places by the necessary exposure of the breast in suckling the child. The invention consists essentially in a nursing attachment designed to be worn over the breast and arranged for the detachable connection thereto of the nipple on a tube of any desired length, the nipple or nipples, according to whether there be one or two employed, being worn inside the shirtwaist or other garment, and it being only necessary when the child is to be nursed, to slip the nipple out of the waist, thereby avoiding the necessity of exposing the person.

So much for man-made technology designed to avoid his, rather than the mother and infant's, embarrassment.

Figure 4.11
Anti-Embarrassment Device

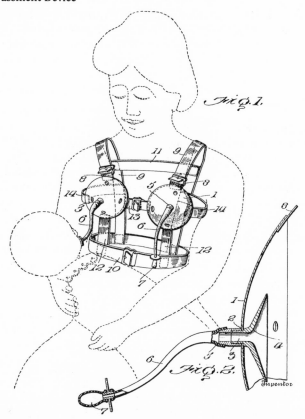

This nursing attachment was "designed to avoid unpleasant and embarrassing situations in which mothers are sometimes placed in public places by the necessary exposure of the breast in suck-ling." *Courtesy*: U.S. Patent Office, Patent No. 949414, 1910. Patented by Hugh Cunningham.

Technological advancements have continued to make bottle-feeding very much simpler than it was. Formula can now be purchased in a variety of forms and sizes. What could be easier than picking up individual servings of ready-to-feed formula in disposable containers? Bottles and teats that function reasonably well are widely available, relatively inexpensive, and easy to clean. Where dishwashers and microwave ovens are available, the preparation of formula and cleaning of baby bottles has become quicker and simpler.

Of course, all this consumer freedom does not come without cost. Not only does the mother miss out on the close bonding of the breastfeeding relationship, not only does the child miss out on the medical advantages breastfed children enjoy, not only must the consumer part with a significant amount of disposable income to acquire the formula and bottles, but there are also compelling and serious environmental implications from artificial feeding.

BOTTLE-FEEDING AND THE ENVIRONMENT

Breastmilk is one of the few foodstuffs which is produced and delivered to the consumer without any pollution, unnecessary packaging or waste. It is the only food which passes on immunization and other health benefits to the consumer and its production also benefits the health of the producer. It is a valuable renewable resource which is usually overlooked. (Andrew Radford, *The Ecological Impact of Bottle Feeding*, 1991)

In this time of increased "green" awareness, more and more efforts are being concentrated on ending depletion of the world's forests, minimizing destruction of the ozone layer, and curtailing contaminants of our soils and seas. Breastfeeding plays a significant role in preserving our environment. The facts below will help illuminate this point.

Substituting Cow's Milk for Breastmilk Is Costly

Formula costs money. It has been estimated that at least $429 million (U.S.) could be saved annually if mothers in the Women, Infants and Children's supplementary feeding program (WIC) would breastfeed for just one month. WIC provides food for pregnant mothers and infants up to three years of age. Formula is by far the most expensive part of the food package and in the last six years costs have risen over 100 percent. WIC accounts for nearly 40 percent of all infant formula purchased in the United States. There are both direct and indirect costs. A tin of powdered formula concentrate in the United States sells for about $10.00. In the first year of life, an infant consumes the contents of approximately seventy cans at a cost of about $700. Liquid concentrates cost more, and ready-to-feed formula costs even more. Add to the formula cost the money spent on bottles, rubber nipples, transportation to buy the formula, and fuel to boil water and clean the bottles. For families who live where tap water is not usable, the cost of bottled water or ready-to-feed formula must also be included.

It would take 135 million lactating cows to substitute for the breastmilk of the women of India. This number of cows would require 43% of the surface area of India for pasture. Land used to grow cattle feed in Third World countries is often land that was formerly used for family food production or land that was forested (deforestation leads to depletion and erosion of soil). Commercial milk production is a very uneconomical use of land. One study determined that producing one kilogram of formula in Mexico costs 12.5 square meters of rain forest. Cow dung and slurry pollutes rivers and ground water, while nitrate fertilizers used to grow feed for dairy cows leach into rivers and ground water.

Artificial Feeding Causes Waste and Uses Valuable Resources

Environmental awareness has increased over the last decade, but few people realize the toll on the environment when breastmilk is withheld. From an ecology point of view, breastmilk could not be greener. Not so for formula. In one year if every child in America were bottle-fed, almost 86,000 tons of tin would be needed to produce 550 million cans of formula wrapped in 1,230 tons of paper labels.

The nation's landfills rise each time a mother does not breastfeed. Formula, of course, has to be put into something in order to get it into the baby. Bottles and nipples require plastic, glass, rubber, and silicon; production of these materials can be resource intensive and often leads to end products that are not recyclable. All these products use natural resources, cause pollution in their manufacture and distribution, and create trash in the packaging, promotion, and disposal.

Once the formula, bottles, and nipples have been brought home, the product has to be prepared. In industrialized countries, this is not particularly hard, but in nonindustrialized nations, this can be quite a production. First, fuel must be found for sterilizing the water and the implements. The majority of people in less developed countries do not have ample access to water. In some parts of Africa, women spend five hours a day just retrieving water (a three-month-old bottle-fed baby needs over three quarts of water a day for boiling and mixing). Fuel to provide heat is equally precious: it takes 200 grams of wood to boil one quart of water. Each bottle-fed baby uses a minimum of seventy-three kilos of valuable wood each year.

Additionally, the average breastfeeding mother goes fourteen months without menstruating if she breastfeeds exclusively. If every mother in Great Britain breastfed, over 3,000 tons of paper would be saved every year just in sanitary protection products. To compound the scenario, breastmilk is absorbed by the baby quite efficiently; breastfed babies excrete less and thus require fewer diaper changes than formula-fed babies. Producing the diapers, menstrual pads, and tampons involves the need for fibers, bleaching, and other chemical processes, packaging materials, fuels used both in manufacturing and product distribution, and, of course, more items to be sent to the landfill.

Breastfeeding Helps Reduce World Population

Breastfeeding is a more effective method of birth control, worldwide, than all other methods available to Third World women. One study of Philippine women whose babies were one year old found that a 20% pregnancy rate for breastfeeding women compared to a 50% pregnancy rate for bottle-feeding women *using* contraception. In Chile, a study of new mothers found no pregnant breastfeeding women at six months postpartum, and a high 72% pregnancy rate at six months postpartum for bottle-feeding women (also see the section on intercourse taboos in chapter 1).

Breastfeeding produces healthier babies in two ways. First, it limits fertility, resulting in greater spacing between births. Infant deaths decrease when spacing is increased. Second, the immunizing agents in breastmilk produce healthier babies and lower the infant death rate. Women have more babies when the infant death rate is high because it is seen as an insurance strategy—more babies increases your chance of at least some of them surviving. But when infant mortality is low, women choose to have fewer children. The effect of breastfeeding on world population is massive. Breastfeeding is credited with preventing an average of 4 births *per woman* in Africa and 6.5 births in Bangladesh. No discussion of how bottle-feeding contributes to depletion of the world's resources is complete without a look at the relationship of bottle-feeding to overpopulation.

While technological advances in both artificial foods and feeding vessels have led to viable alternatives to breastfeeding, it is important to note that all the cases of formula and styles of bottles would still be on the store shelves were it not for aggressive marketing and advertising by the manufacturers. Members of the medical profession and new mothers are routinely targeted for "educational" campaigns promoting the wholesomeness of artificial feeding. Formula companies pass out free samples and coupons to mothers and staff in hospital nurseries—nurseries that, in some instances, were designed, built, and paid for by the formula companies. To complete the cycle, nurses are encouraged to place newborns on formula to facilitate scheduled feedings and central control of nurseries, while mothers are counseled to let the nurses tend to the children so they may catch up on their sleep. To complement the process, literature from formula companies, distributed widely at hospitals, implies that newborn hunger and discontent are common maladies and that bottle-feeding may be part of the solution. From a marketing point of view, this money has been very well spent. A direct correlation between hospital births and a decline in breastfeeding has been clearly documented.

The next chapter describes the way these artificial foods and feeding devices moved from curio to customary, how breastmilk substitutes were transformed from a death sentence to a way of life by an industry that sells, each year, more than $8 billion dollars worth of products, and how women were "taught" that bottle-feeding would liberate them from the confining and unfulfilling role of being a cow and thrust them into modern, liberated motherhood.

Section III

Breastmilk Economics—Shaping Corporate and Governmental Policies

Five

The Global Search for Formula Sales

If your lives were embittered as mine is, by seeing day after day this massacre of the innocents by unsuitable feeding, then I believe you would feel as I do that misguided propaganda on infant feeding should be punished as the most criminal form of sedition, and that these deaths should be regarded as murder.... Anyone who, ignorantly or lightly, causes a baby to be fed on unsuitable milk, may be guilty of that child's death.

—Dr. Cicely D. Williams, "Milk and Murder," 1939

Whereas infant formula companies in the 1800s worked hard to develop formulations that could be used to save the lives of foundlings and sick babies, by the turn of the century, the lure of the global market had become too much. It was no longer the goal to produce a product solely for sick infants or for times when mother's milk was not available; the goal grew to producing a product that could replace mother's milk—on every square inch of the globe.

Skillful marketing and promotion efforts, combined with medical complicity, succeeded in artificial feeding gaining an aura of medical legitimacy. Parents grew to believe that a commercial product could be as good as, or better than, the real thing. By the end of World War II, bottle-feeding had become the standard method of infant feeding in the United States and, to a lesser extent, in Europe as well. With the developed world leading the way, the formula industry expanded their markets by trying to make bottle-feeding the norm in the developing world as well.

The developing world, with its growing populations and rapid urbanization, had relatively weak professional and social institutions and under-staffed government departments. These nations became key targets for the promoters of infant foods. Many developing countries were quite receptive to the arrival of imported artificial milk products. Cases filled with cans of infant formula evoked images of modernization and "keeping up with the West."

Artificial milk also gained legitimacy through international agencies, who were actively distributing free powdered milk. In the early 1960s, the United Nations International Children's Education Fund (UNICEF) was distributing almost two million pounds of milk annually for malnourished infants. This free distribution attracted mothers to clinics, but also gave milk powder the endorsement of health care providers and set the stage for formula marketing in the third world.

In the infant-feeding arena, private profit and public health are at odds. The goals of the baby food industry are in direct conflict with the best interests of babies. For optimal growth and development, a baby's best interests are met when it receives the nutrition and immunologically protective benefits of breastfeeding. The goal of the baby food industry is to maximize its market size by maximizing the number of mothers who buy the products and the length of time they use them. The strategy was to persuade mothers both that breastmilk substitutes and proprietary infant food were more convenient than breastmilk and that mothers may not have sufficient supplies of breastmilk to adequately nourish their children. Through massive marketing efforts and dissemination of often misleading information, infant formula companies succeeded in undermining the confidence of mothers and creating the illusion that artificial products were as good as human breastmilk. The formula industry's strategy included enlisting health care workers, hospitals, and consumers in their marketing (Figure 5.1).

THE SEARCH FOR CONSUMERS

In most low-income countries, breastfeeding is normal in rural areas. Its abandonment is primarily an urban phenomenon. "Urban women could be modern" was the message broadcast into the growing urban areas around the world. Advertising for formula appeared in all the mass media. In countries that had been colonized, bottle-feeding was portrayed as elitism, while breastfeeding became associated with peasantry. Even outside of colonial messages, breastfeeding was associated with peasant women, while bottle-feeding was clearly an activity of the rich and elite.

The bombardment of the formula industry's messages was extensive. Television developed as a new and powerful advertising medium. Billboard advertisements appeared along the roads. Neon signs blinked advertising slogans. Radio messages reached the illiterate. Doctors were given free samples of formula to distribute to their patients, and received in exchange lavish gifts of equipment and research grants.

Figure 5.1
Understanding Marketing

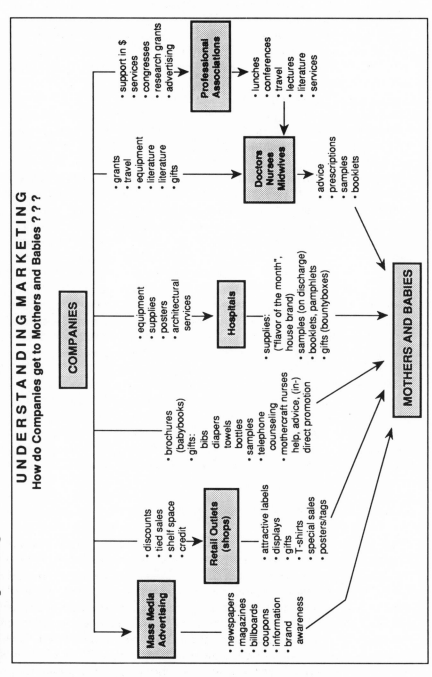
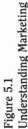

UNDERSTANDING MARKETING
How do Companies get to Mothers and Babies ? ? ?

COMPANIES

Professional Associations
- support in $
- services
- congresses
- research grants
- advertising

- lunches
- conferences
- travel
- lectures
- literature
- services

Doctors
Nurses
Midwives
- grants
- travel
- equipment
- literature
- literature
- gifts

- advice
- prescriptions
- samples
- booklets

Hospitals
- equipment
- supplies
- posters
- architectural services

- supplies: ("flavor of the month", house brand)
- samples (on discharge)
- booklets, pamphlets
- gifts (bountyboxes)

- brochures (babybooks)
- gifts:
  - bibs
  - diapers
  - towels
  - bottles
  - samples
- telephone counseling
- mothercraft nurses help, advice, (in-) direct promotion

Retail Outlets (shops)
- discounts
- tied sales
- shelf space
- credit

- attractive labels
- displays
- gifts
- T-shirts
- special sales
- posters/tags

Mass Media Advertising
- newspapers
- magazines
- billboards
- coupons
- information
- brand awareness

MOTHERS AND BABIES

Source: Janice Mantell, in Breastfeeding: The Passport to Life. Edited by N. Baumslag (New York: UNICEF, 1989).

One particularly insidious marketing technique was the use of "milk nurses." These were women, many of whom were trained nurses, employed by the infant food industries to visit new mothers in hospitals and in their homes in nurses' uniforms to sell formula. They were usually paid on a commission and earned more than a health nurse. One study in Nigeria found that 87% of mothers used artificial milk because they believed they had been advised to do so by hospital staff. The "staff" were, in reality, "milk nurses" allowed into the hospital to ply their wares.

Before this marketing blitz, no one ever doubted the appropriateness of breastmilk. But the only way companies could get women to abandon their long-standing tradition of breastfeeding was to undermine the confidence women had in their own milk. One commercial begged, "When breastmilk fails, choose Lactogen." Other commercials boasted their products had "a cream taste" or high levels of protein and iron. These advertisements made people question the superiority of or even the adequacy of breastmilk. The messages were broadcasted frequently. For example, in August 1974, in Sierra Leone, Sierra Leone Broadcasting Service aired 135 30-second advertisements just for one brand of formula (Nestlé's Lactogen). Lactogen was not the only product competing for the listener's attention. In one month, Unigate also ran forty-five ads for Cow & Gate, while Abbott Laboratories aired sixty-six advertisements for Similac. The advertisements always portrayed the companies as organizations dedicated to providing a sterile, scientific, and superior product for children. They cultivated an image of unquestioning competence, integrity, and backing by the medical profession.

Many mothers started viewing artificial milk as a special food or medicine. They noticed that formula was increasingly used for low-birth-weight and sick infants and began to assume that if it was good for the sick and vulnerable, it was good for healthy infants, too. A new syndrome—"insufficient milk"—began to be diagnosed. Suddenly, large numbers of women didn't have enough milk. And formula sales soared.

PRIVATE PROFIT VERSUS PUBLIC HEALTH

But formula sales were not the only things soaring. Malnutrition and mortality rates also soared as women abandoned breastfeeding. Increasing numbers of infants arrived at hospitals with diarrhea and malnutrition (Figure 5.2). "Bottle-baby disease," the vicious—and often fatal—cycle of diarrhea, dehydration, and malnutrition resulting from unsafe, unhygienic, diluted feeding methods, was increasing in areas where previously the only real breastfeeding problem had been the death of a mother (even in these cases, a relative would breastfeed the orphaned infant). Third-World health workers, international pediatricians, nutritionists, and missionaries grew

Figure 5.2
The Lethal Effect of Formula in Poverty Conditions

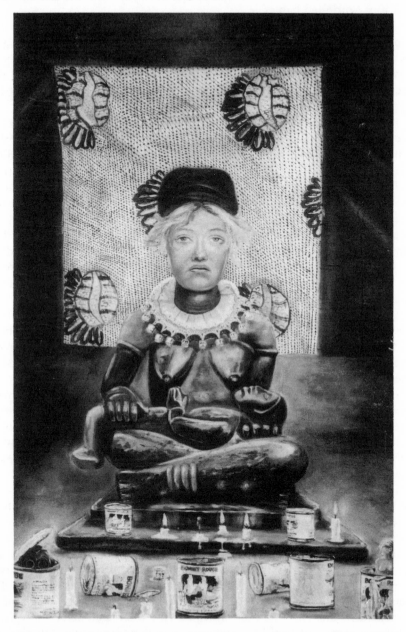

This painting depicts a westernized Congolese mother mourning the death of her baby. The baby was fed infant formula instead of breastmilk. *Source*: *Materna* by Trigo Pivia, Congo. *Photo courtesy*: Museum of African Art, New York, from the exhibition "Africa Explores 20th Century African Art." Photograph by Jerry I. Thompson.

increasingly alarmed at the increase in cases of severe malnutrition and death in bottle-fed babies.

Throughout this century, around the globe, health care professionals found themselves increasingly exasperated at the rising tide of infant malnutrition and death—almost all preventable. Dr. Cicely Williams, a pediatrician working in Singapore in the late 1930s, became so concerned with the high hospital case load and mortality rates that in 1939 she delivered a speech at the Singapore Rotary Club entitled "Milk and Murder" (Figure 5.3). (The chairman of the Rotary Club who presided over the meeting was the local president of Nestlé.) Dr. Williams spoke of "the massacre of the innocents" by unsuitable feeding and urged breastfeeding for the rich and the poor alike.

Ahead of the times, Dr. Williams advocated maternity benefits for poor women workers so they could have adequate time to feed their infants. Her talk caused quite a stir. Not only were her opinions strong, but also her deploring the use of milk substitutes was an about-face, as she had been a proponent of the use of condensed milk for treating *kwashiorkor* (a form of malnutrition) when she worked in Africa. The *Singapore Sun* reported her talk, but it was not published in a medical journal until 1979—when it became more fashionable to promote breastfeeding.

Dr. Williams was joined by other health care workers in subsequent decades in efforts to halt the erosion of breastfeeding. One of these health activists was Dr. Derrick Jelliffe, who coined the term "Commerciogenic Malnutrition" to describe "bottle-baby sickness." Dr. Jelliffe's research in the Caribbean in the 1960s drew attention to the problems caused by bottle-feeding and led to a special meeting sponsored by the Pan American Health Organization (PAHO) in 1970. He presented data that was so impressive that the Jamaican government banned mass media advertising of formula (though the other forms of promotion continued; it took a number of years for concerned health workers and citizens to clearly understand the effectiveness of the industry's insidious marketing strategies).

Dr. Catherine Wennen, a pediatrician from the Netherlands, described similar problems in Nigeria in the 1960s. She was concerned with the increasing numbers of babies sick as a result of bottle-feeding while the radio blared infant formula advertisements and giant billboards beamed photos of healthy bottle-fed babies gleaming with joy. Drs. Puffer and Serrano in Latin America confirmed that the high infant mortality was attributable to bottle-feeding, and Drs. Plank and Milanesi, in Chile, corroborated the connection between bottle-feeding and high infant mortality. Yet the advertisements and sales of infant formula continued unabated.

The warnings of health workers were undermined and ignored as dependence on bottle-feeding increased worldwide. By 1979, a WHO survey found fifty brands and two hundred varieties of infant feeding substitutes being distributed across one hundred countries. All this market success has

Figure 5.3
Milk and Murder

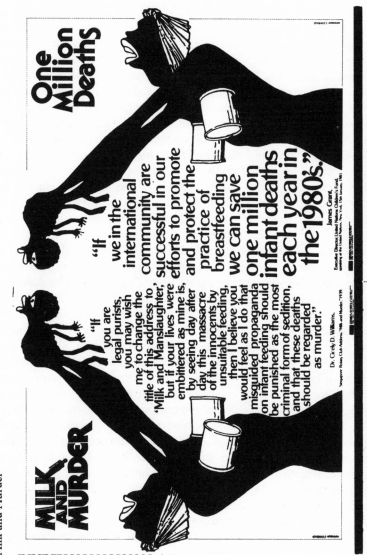

Poster used to create public awareness about the dangers of bottle-feeding. *Photo courtesy:* International Organization of Consumers' Unions, Penang, Malaysia, 1986. Courtesy of UNICEF.

translated into astounding human tragedy. UNICEF estimates that one and a half million babies die each year because they are not breastfed. Most of these deaths are preventable.

TURNING THE TIDE—THE ERA OF ACTIVISM

From the early 1970s, the tide began to turn. The collective, concerned voices of health care workers and activists around the world finally became audible enough to result in the United Nations Protein Advisory Group meeting to discuss the problem. But when industry representatives were confronted with the consequences of their indiscriminate sales promotions, they insisted that advertising did not really influence people, it simply made consumers aware of their choices. They asserted that people do not buy what they do not need, and that therefore the industry bore no responsibility for the consequences of the market penetration.

Broader awareness of the problem finally came in 1973, via the *New Internationalist*, a British publication that ran an interview with David Morley and Ralph Hendrikse, two pediatricians who had worked in Africa. They described the problem in everyday language. Then, in 1974, the British charity, War on Want, published *The Baby Killer*, in which journalist Mike Muller wrote a dramatic account of the tactics (and the results) used by formula companies to capture the market (Figure 5.4). *The Baby Killer* had a powerful cover picture, as well as tragic pictures of impoverished, malnourished infants. It was widely translated and distributed. Other reports and studies followed, including a critical *Consumer's Union* investigation of food and pharmaceutical industries by Robert Ledogar and a book, *The Nutrition Factor*, by The Brookings' Institute scholar Alan Berg. This spurred WHO in 1974 to call for a review of corporate sales practices and to advise member governments to consider action.

In 1975, *Bottle Babies*, a documentary by Peter Krieg, was released. Filmed in Kenya, it was filled with powerful visual images of starving, malnourished, bottle-fed infants. In one scene, a mother was shown scooping water from a filthy pool and mixing it with baby formula. In another scene, a graveyard marked by bottles and formula cans (the prized possessions) were also shown; there, as in other parts of the world, it is customary to bury the most valued possession with the infant (Figure 5.5). The film created a ground swell of activity to curb inappropriate promotion of infant foods and proved to be an effective tool for making many people aware of the problems created by bottle-feeding.

In the meantime, a Swiss Third World Action Group, called Arbeitsgruppe Dritte Welt (AgDW), translated *The Baby Killer* into German and retitled it provocatively *Nestlé Kills Babies*. This sparked a wave of worldwide publicity as well as a libel suit against the group by Nestlé. Two days

Figure 5.4
"The Baby Killer"

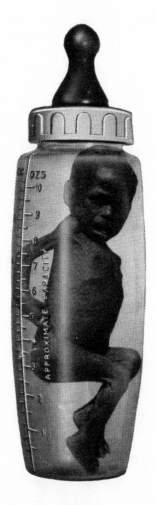

Cover image of *The Baby Killer*. *Source*: Andy Chetley, *War on Want Report*, United Kingdom, 1974. *Photo courtesy*: War on Want.

before the trial officially opened, formula manufacturers announced the creation of the International Council of Infant Formula Industries (ICIFI) to improve their image. ICIFI announced that it was preparing a code of ethics for infant formula companies. At the final hearing of the libel case in March 1976, the judge ruled that, since it could not be shown that

Figure 5.5
Modern Marketing Killed This Baby

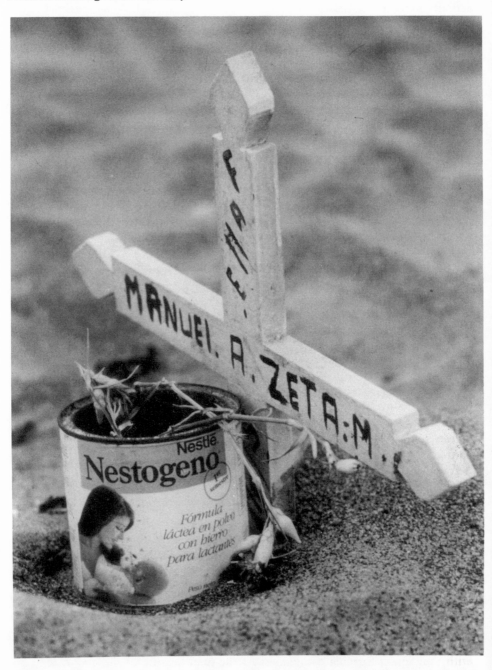

The grave of a victim of bottle-baby disease in Chimbote, Peru. *Photo courtesy*: Christian Aid, courtesy of Baby Milk Action.

Nestlé's sales practices *directly* killed infants (as the mother is the one who actually prepares the bottle), the title of the article by AgDW was technically libelous and imposed a token fine on them. The judge sternly stated, however, that it was not an acquittal and that Nestlé must "fundamentally rethink" its advertising practices if it wanted to be spared the accusation of immoral and unethical conduct. It was considered a great victory for the fledgling campaign created to curtail the activities of the formula companies.

Throughout the 1970s, outrage against formula companies grew. The trial in Switzerland sparked a chain reaction of events in the United States. American church groups concerned with world hunger and social responsibility filed stockholder resolutions with American companies in which they owned stock, requesting information on international sales practices. Stockholder actions were directed at Bristol Myers (producer of Enfamil) and coordinated through the Interfaith Center for Social Responsibility; the Sisters of Precious Blood in Dayton, in particular, generated an enormous amount of bad publicity about Bristol Myers. Finally, in 1978, Bristol Myers agreed to halt mass media advertising and to take their milk nurses out of Jamaica, where they had been soliciting business in a public hospital.

Concerned shareholders of other companies also resolved to end unethical sales promotion of formula in areas where people lacked the means to bottle-feed safely. Borden, another U.S. formula company, agreed to stop advertising Klim as an infant food, and Abbott agreed to take "mothercraft nurses" out of uniform. But Nestlé, the world leader in baby milk sales, continued to dominate the baby milk market and to engage in aggressive promotion. *Fortune Magazine* estimated that, in 1977, Nestlé was the most profitable food company in the world. And U.S. citizens could not use investor influence, as only Swiss nationals could own shares in the company.

A consumer organization called the Infant Formula Action Coalition (INFACT) was formed, with headquarters in Minnesota, to monitor formula companies, circulate the findings, and lobby for change. In 1977, INFACT initiated a consumer boycott against Nestlé (Figure 5.6). The aim of the boycott was to force Nestlé to end practices detrimental to breastfeeding. INFACT demanded that Nestlé halt all promotion of baby milk, including milk nurses, free samples, and advertising. The film *Bottle Babies* was shown all over the United States to publicize the lethal effect of formula in developing countries. This was followed in 1978 by a letter-writing campaign on the problem of formula abuse in the third world; letters were sent to Nestlé at an estimated rate of 400 a week. The boycott received tremendous support from church groups, many of whom had direct contact with the developing countries through their missionary work and were in a position to verify facts of the marketing abuses. The boycott gained mo-

Figure 5.6
Boycott Poster

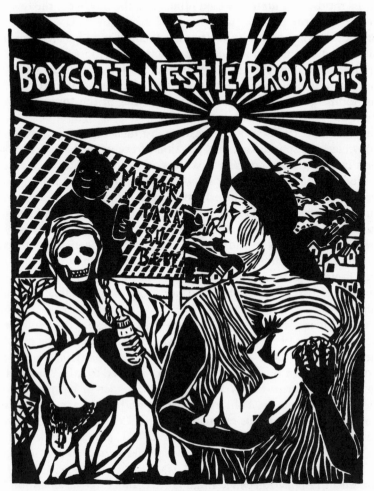

This poster was circulated widely to rally support for the Nestlé boycott. *Source*:
Unknown.

mentum in the United States and quickly spread to Canada, Europe, and New Zealand.

Fearing the effect on its sales, Nestlé held its ground and invested in an aggressive campaign to restore its image. The company contracted with the public relations firm of Hill & Knowlton to develop and distribute hundreds of thousands of glossy booklets defending themselves to clergy and religious bodies. They insisted that Nestlé did not aggressively market baby milk in the third world. That campaign alone cost $1 million.

While executives at Nestlé were receiving outraged letters from the public, so, too, were members of the U.S. Congress. As the issue initiated more discussion in the media, and as pressure from concerned health care workers and nutritionists increased, Congress launched its own investigation. Senator Edward Kennedy, chairman of the Subcommittee on Health and Scientific Research, held a hearing in 1978 on the promotion and use of infant formula in developing countries. The hearings were packed with reporters and became the first major exposure of the issue to policy makers and the national media.

Senator Kennedy opened the hearing by saying; "It is astonishing, and it is an enormous tragedy, that one-fourth of the people on this earth—one billion men, women, and children—have no access to any health care whatsoever . . . and it is always the children who suffer most." He went on to ask the witnesses a key question: "Can a product which requires clean water, good sanitation, adequate family income, and a literate parent to follow printed instructions, be properly and safely used in areas where water is contaminated, sewage runs in the streets, poverty is severe, and illiteracy high?" He also asked, "Whose responsibility is it . . . when economic incentives are in conflict with public health requirements [and] how shall the conflict be resolved?"

At the hearing, there were three panels of witnesses who presented testimony. The first was a panel of missionaries, doctors, and church activists who worked in developing countries and had firsthand knowledge of the practices that cause poor mothers to bottle-feed. They were followed by a panel of distinguished physicians and health experts who were unanimous in their concern about the decline in breastfeeding and the rise of bottle-feeding with its associated illnesses. They were unequivocal that industry sales tactics played a key role in creating this situation. The hearings showed that the advertising and marketing of infant formula had penetrated into the most remote regions of developing countries. One witness testified that formula was sold in a tribal area of the Amazon region accessible only by foot or light plane. It was at these hearings that Dr. Jelliffe stated that even cans of puppy formula contain a warning that it should not be given in the first days of life so that puppies may obtain the anti-infective benefits of colostrum (the initial breastmilk). He pointed out this warning was wholly absent on cans of formula for humans. Many witnesses cited the detrimental consequences that result when infant formula is improperly diluted (a phenomenon known as "stretching") and used by mothers to make formula last longer.

The most dramatic testimony of the day was that of Dr. Natividad Clavano, Chief of Pediatrics at Baguio General Hospital in the Philippines, who described how the hospital had successfully addressed the infant formula problem by refusing to allow the milk nurses access to new mothers, removing formula promotion posters, ending the distribution of formula samples, instituting immediate breastfeeding after birth, and twenty-four-hour-a-day rooming in. In just over four years, in a population of 10,000 infants, the breastfeeding rate jumped from 26% to 87%. Furthermore, Dr. Clavano stated, "we were able to reduce our infant deaths by over 47% and diseases by 58%. Diarrhea was reduced by 79%." In the place of formula company posters, they hung reproductions of the cover of *The Baby Killer*.

The third panel consisted of the representatives of formula companies who maintained that their own Code of Ethics was sufficient to prevent abuse. Nonetheless, both the Nestlé and Wyeth representatives were forced to concede that their products were readily available to the poor in developing countries, and that they were either unable or unwilling to do anything about it. At one point in the hearing, Senator Kennedy questioned Oswaldo Ballerin, President of Nestlé Brazil, as to whether his company should market a product in areas without clean water and where people were illiterate. Ballerin first declared that all instructions were on the can. When pressed, he responded, "But . . . we cannot be responsible for that." After further questioning, Ballerin stated, "The U.S. Nestlé Company has advised me that their research indicates that this [boycott] is actually an indirect attack on the free world's economic system. A world-wide church organization, with the stated purpose of undermining the free enterprise system, is in the forefront of this activity." These comments were met with raucous laughter.

The Kennedy hearings were a turning point for the whole reform movement. They enhanced the credibility of industry critics and helped propel the Nestlé boycott to a wider base of support. It also mobilized a number of major institutions to address the problem and find some solutions, and led to the convening of the WHO/UNICEF Meeting on Infant and Young Child Feeding in October 1979 in Geneva, Switzerland. This was welcomed by everyone involved in the controversy. Nestlé pledged to abide by anything the meeting decided and tried, with some success, to head off boycott endorsements by making such promises.

However, the tenacity and reach of the industry was not to be minimized. Shortly after the Kennedy hearings, an International Nutrition Congress was held in Rio de Janeiro. The major sponsors were Nestlé and Coca Cola. The Nestlé's corporate logo adorned name badges and meeting paraphernalia, and their consumer products were on view and highly publicized. Media Benjamina, a conference participant and former Food and Agriculture Organization staffer, circulated a petition criticizing Nestlé for promoting infant formula in the third world. She was arrested and detained by plain-clothes Brazilian security police; her "crime" appears to have been circulation of the petition. Two top-level U.S. officials had to intervene. After her release, she was quickly sent back to the United States disguised in men's clothing. In a display of editorial courage, Brazil's leading newspaper denounced the arrest as an illegal assault on the civil liberties of a foreigner. This story helps illustrate how hard it is for committed health workers to stand up against such corporate might.

DEVELOPING THE WHO CODE

The WHO/UNICEF meeting on the International Code of Marketing of Breastmilk Substitutes was unusual not only because of the controversy but also because one hundred and fifty selected governments, international experts, and industry and consumer groups were given individual participant status. The meeting set as its goal the development of a joint statement to improve child nutrition and properly support breastfeeding through health services. A document was produced whose key points were: no sales promotion to the public of products used as breastmilk substitutes, information given by health personnel should be only factual and ethical, and an international code of marketing for infant formula should be developed. It was agreed that this the statement developed should be supported by both exporting and importing countries and observed by all manufacturers. WHO/UNICEF were then requested to organize the process for preparation of such a Code, as soon as possible, with the involvement of all concerned parties.

Dr. Mahler, the World Health Director, concluded the meeting with the following statement: "In my opinion, the campaign against bottle-feed advertising is unbelievably more important than the fight against smoking advertisement. . . . [T]here is no way the infant food industry can get away with what they have been doing in the past and say they have our stamp of approval."

Nestlé and ICIFI immediately pledged to abide by the recommendations. Nestlé sent mailings to hundreds of thousands of Americans to announce their new position. "Nestlé and the industry of which it is a part completely support the statement of WHO/UNICEF." The statement was also endorsed by the governing boards of both WHO and UNICEF as well as by the American Medical Association (AMA) and the American Academy of Pediatrics (AAP). Meanwhile, consumer groups from every continent

banded together to monitor industry compliance with "the recommendations," calling itself the International Baby Food Action Network (IBFAN).

But soon after the meeting, Nestlé president Arthur Furer told a Swiss
newspaper, "We feel in no way restricted in our commercial activities by
the recommendations of WHO." And under questioning by a subcommittee
of the House of Representatives in February 1980, neither Nestlé nor any
of the three American companies (Abbott Laboratories, American Home
Products, and Bristol Meyers) were able to list the changes they planned
to make. In 1980 alone, IBFAN documented 682 industry violations of the
recommendations.

In May 1980, the World Health Assembly (WHA), the annual assembly
of member nations of WHO, voted to ask the Secretariat to draft a Code
and oversee international discussion as called for in the 1979 recommendations. During the following year, there were four draft Codes and numerous "consultations" on each draft with all parties. All the companies
said they were cooperating with the Code process and supported the development of a Code, but they continued to work behind the scenes to
oppose the Code and discredit the industry critics. An article was distributed that claimed that religious supporters of the Nestlé Boycott were
"Marxists marching under the banner of Christ." Bristol Myers mailed
80,000 copies of the article to shareholders; it was also distributed to a list
of "opinion leaders." While Nestlé stated adamantly that the boycott was
not harming their business, their public relations efforts suggested otherwise.

In January 1981, ICIFI President Ernest Saunders declared that the fourth
(and final) draft of the Code was "unacceptable," then two months later
said "ICIFI members continue to support the statement and recommendations of the October 1979 meeting." During this period, the U.S. government had been developing its position. An "Interagency Task Force" of key
government representatives weighed the issues and was generally pro-Code
during the Carter Administration. However, the issue was revisited by the
Reagan Administration when the White House changed hands in 1981.
Meanwhile, American industry came out publicly and forcefully against the
Code in March. They called it "a set of highly specific and restrictive rules
that would virtually eliminate legitimate competition and promotion of infant formula even to the medical community." Nestlé lobbied heavily
against the Code everywhere in the world.

In May 1981, the WHA convened in Geneva to vote on the WHO/
UNICEF Code of Marketing of Breastmilk Substitutes. It was overwhelmingly approved by 118 countries. There were three abstentions; the U.S.
delegate, Dr. John Bryant, under orders from the State Department, reluc-
tantly cast the only opposing vote. The U.S. position was met with shock
and dismay at home and abroad. Two leading officials of the U.S. Agency
for International Development (USAID) who were members of the U.S.
delegation to the 1991 WHO meeting, Dr. Steve Joseph and Tony Babb,

resigned in protest. The White House and State Department received 10,000 letters and telegrams. The public outcry was so great that both the House of Representatives and the Senate overwhelmingly approved resolutions expressing dismay at the vote (the House passed it 301–100, the Senate 89–2). Although the language of the resolution was mild, the political sentiment was clear, as liberals and conservatives of both parties spoke out strongly in the floor debate. Newspaper editorials in U.S. papers disagreed with the U.S. vote by more than 4–1, using words like "shameful," "callous," and "inhumane." U.S. supporters of the Code called for a mock wake outside the White House to symbolize that health professionals and the public were against the U.S. vote.

The U.S. government's decision to vote against the Code was the result of an extensive lobbying effort by the baby food corporations of the Reagan Administration. The decision was made by four top administration officials: Ed Meese, Lyn Nofziger, Martin Anderson, and Richard Allen. These men overruled the opinions of the country's highest health officials. The pretext for the U.S. vote was that the Code put unnecessary burdens on corporations in a political climate focused on getting government out of the corporate suites, noting that the infant formula industry represented a $2-billion-and-growing international market (it has since more than tripled). They acquiesced to fears that adoption of the Code would set a precedent that might lead to action in other fields like pharmaceuticals. They even convinced politicians that provisions in the voluntary Code would cause constitutional problems for the United States itself (a concern for which there was no basis).

Despite the extraordinary public outcry when the administration decision became known *prior* to the vote, President Reagan repeatedly refused to meet with a bipartisan Congressional delegation that sought to change his mind. Representative Tom Harkin was told that the President had no time on his schedule. Harkin told newspaper columnist Judy Mann, "I cannot believe the President can't find ten minutes in the day to meet with 12–15 members of Congress on an issue of this importance. I know how tight a President's schedule is, but . . . I don't want to see the President to give him a ten-gallon hat or to declare June 15 National Tulip Day. This is something much more important."

Though the United States only has one vote, it still dominates the world economy and establishes political priorities. When the United States voted to put profit making above human welfare, it sent a message that strict enforcement of the Code was not required.

THE CODE

The WHO/UNICEF Code of Marketing of Breastmilk Substitutes (the WHO Code) is the first international consumer code—albeit a voluntary

Table 5.1
The WHO/UNICEF International Code of Marketing of Breastmilk Substitutes

---

The aim of the Code is:

. . . to contribute to the provision of safe and adequate nutrition for infants, by the protection and promotion of breastfeeding and by the proper use of breastmilk substitutes, when these are necessary, on the basis of adequate information and through appropriate marketing and distribution.

The Code includes ten main provisions:

1.   No advertising of breastmilk substitutes.

2.   No free samples of breastmilk substitutes to mothers.

3.   No promotion of products through health care facilities.

4.   No company mothercraft nurses to advise mothers.

5.   No gifts or personal samples to health workers.

6.   No words or pictures idealizing artificial feeding, including pictures of infants, on the labels of the products.

7.   Information to health workers should be scientific and factual.

8.   All information on artificial feeding, including the labels, should explain the benefits of breastfeeding and the costs and hazards associated with artificial feeding.

9.   Unsuitable products, such as sweetened condensed milk, should not be promoted for babies.

10. All products should be of a high quality and take into account the climatic and storage conditions of the country where they are used.

Source: WHO/UNICEF, The WHO/UNICEF International Code of Marketing of Breastmilk Substitutes, adopted in Geneva, Switzerland, May 1981.

one. It is an international standard, not an international law. Politics and rhetoric aside, the Code is really a simple document that recommends that member governments restrict advertising and sales promotions of breastmilk substitutes. Each nation is free to adapt the Code (Table 5.1) within the national and legal frameworks of its own society. It was adopted as a "minimum requirement" to protect infant health.

The Code does not restrict the availability or sale of formula or any other product. Rather, it seeks to end the glamorization of artificial feeding and to prevent the product from being used unnecessarily by those who will not be able to afford it and/or use it safely. No coercion can be brought to bear on any country to implement the Code. It is similar to international rules governing sporting events whereby nations agree on rules and policies governing international competitions. *Asia Week* magazine, reflecting what was the clear sentiment of the world community, said that the Code, "approved by a gathering of nations, both rich and poor," is "perhaps the most significant international consumer protection standard of modern times."

Figure 5.7
Excerpt from a UNICEF-Sponsored Booklet

Describing one Nestlé milk nurse, the booklet states:

*He seems to be everywhere at the same time—at clinics in remote rural areas, at health
education programmes and at conferences (where he . . . sometimes takes health workers
out for meals). Wherever he goes, he leaves a Nestlé trail behind him, in the form of free
samples, Nestlé calendars for the wall and for the desk, Nestlé "Road to Health" cards
and "informative" material.*

*The charm and the appearance of genuine concern . . . that dress up these activities only
serve to promote the gain of the Food Specialties (Nestlé) Company—at the expense of
the Zimbabwean people.*

Source: Baby-Feeding: Behind and Towards a Health Model for Zimbabwe (Harare: Zimbabwe Ministry of Health, 1981). *Courtesy:* UNICEF.

Adoption of the Code in Geneva was one thing, implementation was
another. Nonetheless, the Code has had a number of positive effects, including the promotion of breastfeeding on a larger scale and an increased
awareness by health workers of the problems of bottle-feeding.

THE BOYCOTT ENDS . . . AND BEGINS AGAIN

Even after adoption of the Code, Nestlé still took little action to change
their marketing practices, so the boycott continued and strengthened. Nestlé distributors in Zimbabwe went so far as to try and stop publication of
a UNICEF-sponsored breastfeeding booklet for health workers, *Baby Feeding: Behind and Towards a Health Model for Zimbabwe,* which was published in 1981 by the Ministry of Health. Distribution was stalled while
Nestlé representatives approached the Zimbabwe's Attorney General's office to postpone the publication. Mr. Schaepper, Nestlé's Managing Director in Harari, said the booklet "is polemical and destructive."

What was in the booklet that was "polemical and destructive"? It warned
against the dangers of bottle-feeding and promoted breastfeeding. It included a section of quotes from health workers on the aggressive sales
campaign of Nestlé, especially in the rural areas (Figure 5.7). It documented
the milk nurses' tactics, free samples, calendars, posters, promotional booklets, and weight cards as Nestlé's prime marketing techniques. It told mothers how to breastfeed, discussed the problems with bottle-feeding,
explained the WHO/UNICEF Code, and outlined steps to encourage breastfeeding. Despite the pressure to block its distribution, the booklet was finally released in January 1982.

Nestlé continued to assert that the boycott was not hurting them economically, but according to Swiss journalist Jean-Claude Buffle, it cost Nestlé over $1.1 billion. After the passage of the WHO/UNICEF International Code of Marketing of Breastmilk Substitutes in 1981, Nestlé stated that it would direct its employees to abide by this Code. Later, Nestlé signed an agreement with the International Nestlé Boycott Committee in which they agreed to develop marketing policies that were consistent with the intent of the Code and to follow guidelines to be established by UNICEF and WHO on the distribution of free supplies. As a result, the boycott was suspended in early 1984, and after a six-month test period, it was officially halted and declared a success.

However, curtailing the boycott seemed only to give Nestlé license to continue on its path of rapid market expansion. In response to continuing widespread and egregious violations of the International Code, Action for Corporate Accountability reinstated the boycott against Nestlé in October 1988. The International Nestlé Boycott Committee now has coordinating groups in fourteen countries, with millions of individuals in seventy countries participating. The boycott was also expanded to target American Home Products (the second largest manufacturer of infant formula in the world) by groups in the United States, Philippines, Australia, and Canada. Backers of the boycott vow it will continue this time until sustained monitoring shows that these two companies have ended all their promotion of bottle-feeding. The boycott is actively supported by the Church of England, the Swedish Church, and the General Synod of the Anglican Church of Canada (more information on the boycott can be found in Appendix D).

IS THE CODE WORKING?

More than a decade has passed since the Code was ratified. Within three years of the Code's adoption, 130 countries had taken some form of action on it. Some countries have brought in the Code as a voluntary measure, though only nine countries have introduced it as national law. Various excuses have been given, such as incompatibility with national constitutions, low priority, or interference by the baby milk industry. Over the last decade, the steady downward breastfeeding rates have begun to reverse. Public health officials, health organizations, and medical professionals have worked together to counter the bottle-feeding trend. Today, in Finland and Sweden, 95% of babies are breastfed from birth (Table 5.2); in Germany, almost 70% of babies are breastfed at two months.

Some areas of improvement can be seen, notably in labeling and advertising; however, compliance by industry has been pitiful and violations are rampant. Monitoring is difficult. IBFAN accumulates reports of violations and produces *Breaking the Rules*, a worldwide report on violations of the Code, indexed both by company and country. The report cites such violations as an advertisement in Saudi Arabia stating that Nan formula "pro-

Table 5.2
Factors That Help Boost Breastfeeding Rates: The Scandinavian Experience

---

Throughout the 1970s and 1980s, the breastfeeding rate in Scandinavia rose from 30% to nearly 90% for infants three months old. Some of the factors behind this rise included:

- producing problem-based information, written by and for mothers

- expanding mother-to-mother support nationally, which led to an increased positive experience for health workers

- maternity leave was prolonged for one year

- maternity ward practices changed to more mother-infant contact and autonomy

- formula companies maintained a low profile (as the market was small)

- a growing and vocal feminist movement

- high acceptance of the exposure of breasts (largely stemming from the relaxed Swedish attitude toward the body and the tradition of women sunbathing topless)

Source: E. Helsing, "Supporting Breastfeeding: What Government and Health Workers Can Do. European Experience." In *Breastfeeding: Passport to Life*, edited by N. Baumslag (New York: NGO Committee on UNICEF, Working Group on Nutrition, 1989).

motes the same physiological characteristics in all important parameters as in breastfed infants"; American Home Products, Wyeth-Ayerst Laboratories (Appendix E) gives free supplies to at least twenty-five developing countries and seven developed nations; in Point-à-Pierre hospitals in San Fernando, Trinidad, and Tobago, every baby born is fed on free supplies of S-26 from Wyeth; no baby is breastfed and all mothers receive a sample can at hospital discharge; Nestlé still gives away free supplies of baby milk to at least forty-five developing countries and ten developed nations.

IBFAN also found that the baby milk industry has spent a good amount of effort devising ways to appear to be in compliance with the Code while making maximum use of gray areas. One such area involves getting around restrictions on free samples. In the Netherlands, the Catharina Hospital in Eindhoven buys the baby milk it uses—Nutricia's Almiron m2—and the hospital receives an annual "cooperation fee" from Nutricia. Not surprisingly, the fee increases as the hospital purchases increase. Free samples are distributed to every mother, resulting in nearly 90% of babies being on mixed feeding before hospital discharge.

Another such area of violation of the Code involves "follow-up" milks, that is, infant formula marketed for infants six months and older. These were practically nonexistent when the Code was drafted. Now, nearly every company has launched at least one of these milk types in an attempt to widen the market and evade Code restrictions. Companies claim they are not breastmilk substitutes and therefore are exempt from marketing restrictions. The label designs and names of the follow-up milks are often the same as the producer's standard infant formula, simply with the addition of "II" or "plus." The fact that they are infant foods, given in bottles, with all the dangers of bottle-feeding, takes advantage of the fact that the Code does not specifically restrict advertising of "follow-up" milk.

Yet another scheme to avoid restrictions imposed by the Code is practiced in Switzerland. Baby milk manufacturer Milupa sends a letter to new mothers promoting Milactin, a tea for mothers that purports to aid breastfeeding. The letter contains information suggesting mothers need such aids to successfully breastfeed and offers free samples of their infant formula. Mothers requesting tea samples also receive baby milk samples, even if they do not request them.

To market their products, companies still could give donations of breastmilk substitutes to hospitals and health centers. To close this loophole in the Code, the 1986 WHO Assembly in May passed a resolution urging the banning of donations of breastmilk substitutes in all maternity hospitals. This was passed by ninty-two countries, with six abstentions; once again, the United States cast the only vote of opposition. Dr. E. Maganu of the Ministry of Health, Botswana, in support of banning donations of breastmilk substitutes, stated at the 1986 World Health Assembly, "There comes a point when compromise for the sake of consensus becomes surrender. Our babies are the ones who suffer if these marketing practices continue. When there is a conflict between infant health and commercial practices, it is the practices which must stop. These milk donations harm our babies by discouraging breastfeeding, the best, safest way to feed infants."

Furthermore, the Assembly noted that, "Only small quantities of breastmilk substitutes are ordinarily required to meet the needs of a minority of infants . . . and they should only be available in ways that do not interfere with the protection and promotion of breastfeeding for the majority." To combat misinterpretations of the Code, specific guidelines recommended under which circumstances infants would have to be fed on breastmilk substitutes. The guidelines adopted recommend that breastfeeding be discontinued only for specific situations such as inherited metabolic disorders of the infant, if the mother is critically ill, or in times of acute social disruption such as famine, war, or earthquake. The immunological, nutritional, and emotional advantages of breastfeeding, especially during the first months, are still considered to outweigh risks associated with modern life, such as exposure to infectious diseases, foreign chemical compounds, and environmental contaminants such as PCBs.

The struggle continues as companies vie for customers and make new products. According to IBFAN, Nestlé violated twenty-two sections of the Code in fifty-six countries just in 1990 and 1991. AHP violated twenty sections of the Code in thirty-five countries during the same two years. Though some improvements have been made, the companies are still violating almost every section of the Code. For instance, Nestlé took hundreds of Brazilian pediatricians on a nine-day luxury cruise in 1993, and advertises on U.S. Television (which is also against guidelines of the American Academy of Pediatrics).

Free supplies of artificial baby milks are still a widespread, serious problem. Informational materials produced by the formula companies continue to be promotional, and all the companies continue to give a wide range of gifts to health workers. Improvements have been made in labeling, but Gerber, Snow, and Wyeth still have pictures of babies on some of their labels. Not a single infant formula company today can demonstrate full compliance with the Code.

THE UNITED STATES EMBRACES THE CODE

The concern for markets of multinational corporations must never again outweigh the health of the world's infants. (Karlyn Sturmer, Action for Corporate Accountability, 1994)

Compliance with the Code may very well improve dramatically in the latter half of the 1990s, because the United States just reversed its thirteen years of isolated opposition to the Code (and all previous resolutions). On May 9, 1994, signaling a tremendous policy shift, President Clinton made the World Health Organization's International Code of Marketing of Breastmilk Substitutes worldwide policy by joining with the other member nations at the World Health Assembly in Geneva. For the first time, there is worldwide unanimity that, in the infant health arena, profit should not come before public health. World Health Resolution 47.5 (Table 5.3) took a long time in coming, but supporters of the Code say it is the welcome completion of the work begun in 1978 when the Kennedy hearings exposed the industry's role in bottle-baby deaths and led to the effort to develop a Code.

Lobbying on both sides of the issue was strong, with the International Association of Infant Formula Manufacturers (IFM) and American Home Products circulating to key U.S. State Department and Health and Human Services officials amendments that would severely weaken the resolution and the Code. A task force of breastfeeding proponents, including representatives from the U.S. Committee for UNICEF, the La Leche League, UNICEF, and the American Public Health Association, made passage of the amendment their focus for months leading up to the vote. Providing high-profile endorsements were former President Jimmy Carter, Drs. Benjamin Spock and C. Everett Koop, Senator Kennedy, UNICEF Executive Director James Grant, and national consumer leader Ralph Nader. Melinda Kimbell, deputy assistant secretary at the State Department, indicated that

Table 5.3
World Health Resolution 47.5

At the World Health Assembly Meeting in Geneva in May 1994, the United States reversed its lone opposition to the WHO/UNICEF International Code of Marketing of Breastmilk Substitutes. The Code was adopted by international consensus. Here is a summary of what was gained:

1. In theory, the United States is now in support of the Code. The door is open at last for the United States to do what the Code calls for: "to take action appropriate to [its] social and legislative framework and [its] overall development objectives to give effect to the principles and aim of this Code, including the enactment of legislation, regulations or other suitable measures."

2. WHA Resolution 47.5 clarifies Resolution 39.28 (passed in 1986) and affirms that all products under the scope of the Code, not just infant formula, are not to be provided for free or at subsidized cost. It states that this is intended for *the whole health care system*, not just maternity wards and maternity hospitals. This language closes significant loopholes claimed by the industry.

3. WHA 47.5 also corroborates the position of the health care community that most babies need *no other food* than breastmilk *until the age of about six months* and also emphasizes the need for local foods—not expensive, imported, processed foods or follow-up milks—and continued breastfeeding.

Source: *Action News*, Action for Corporate Accountability (Summer 1994).

Secretary Warren Christopher was moved by the hundreds of individualized letters he received from health workers, parents, and activists on the issue.

Acrimonious debate over industry-sponsored amendments ensued for three days. The United States, Italy, and Ireland attempted to champion the industry-backed amendments. Fortunately, the African nations, strongly united in a block, vehemently opposed the presumption that they needed donations from baby milk companies. In fact, the Swaziland delegation, speaking for the African nations (including South Africa, for the first time in thirty years), countered the industry initiative by proposing to strengthen the resolution even more. Kenya demanded that if the issue came to a vote, it would insist on a roll call of member states "so that those who are unfair to babies would be known by name." One by one, all countries agreed to withdraw amendments and expressed support for the resolution. In a dramatic moment, the chair declared that WHA Resolution 47.5 had been approved by full consensus. Nearly universal applause filled the chamber. Hopefully, a new area of cooperation has begun.

THE MEDICAL CONNECTION

Infant formula is a concoction of either cow's milk or soya milk with vitamins and other nutrients. The precise ingredients are prescribed by law. Yet infant formula sales are astoundingly profitable. A sixteen-ounce can of formula in Washington, DC, costs just under $10. When reconstituted, it will make fifteen eight-ounce bottles, which is about a two-day supply for a four-month-old baby. Over a year, it adds up to about $1,800 (the actual cost of formula feeding is, of course, higher when you add in the bottles, nipples, water, and fuel). This represents not only a significant burden on the families but also represents a significant windfall for the manufacturers. Florida's Attorney General calculated that for every dollar the formula company charges for wholesale baby milk, only 16¢ is spent on production and delivery. With such a large spread between cost and sales price, it's easy to see how Abbott Laboratories (whose Similac brand holds 51% of the U.S. formula market) has been able to post 15% profit increases every year for over two decades, and how infant formula sales comprise up to 50% of the *total* profits of Abbott Labs, an enormous pharmaceutical concern.

Where is all that money going? It is not going to help poor and sick children. It is going to subsidize formula costs in third-world countries. It is going into the pockets of the industry executives. As reported in *The Washington Post*, the chief executive of Bristol Myers (makers of Enfamil) earns a whopping annual salary of $12,788,000. The chief executive at Abbott Laboratories (makers of Similac) takes home much less—only $4,213,000 a year!

The companies would like us to believe that they are willing to share the wealth; after all, they have been more than generous in supporting and lavishing gifts on medical professionals and organizations. The professional health bodies (which have the responsibility of reporting Code violations) frequently receive funding for salaries, grants, and conferences from the major manufacturers. The formula makers contribute about $1 million annually to the American Academy of Pediatrics (AAP) in the form of a renewable grant; the grant has already netted the AAP $8 million. The industry also kicked in at least $3 million toward the cost of building the Academy's headquarters in Illinois in 1983. At the AAP's biannual meetings, formula companies routinely pay for parties and receptions.

In 1993, the American College of Obstetrics and Gynecologists (ACOG) received $236,000 from Mead Johnson (of Enfamil fame) and $312,000 from Wyeth-Ayerst (of SMA fame). Wyeth-Ayerst and Abbott Laboratories (of Similac fame) underwrite the American Medical Association (AMA) television program. All three of these formula companies advertise in the journals of the AAP, the AMA, and ACOG. (Appendix E lists the companies that sell formula in the United States and which brands they sell.) Other groups accepting financial support from the formula companies include the Association of Women's Health, Obstetric, and Neonatal Nurses; the American Dietetic Association; and the National Association of Neonatal Nurses. (UNICEF particularly opposes formula company grants that underwrite activities related to breastfeeding, such as "educational" programs for a hospital's personnel.)

Individuals also benefit handsomely from a relationship with industry. Formula makers have extended benefits to medical students and pediatricians; these include school loans, grants, payments for articles, gifts, and trips to conferences. An increasing proportion of medical and nutrition research is financed by baby milk companies. Outright cash grants in the thousands of dollars have been given to physicians who recommend specific products. All sides earnestly claim there are no strings attached, but more often than not, the recipients of company money are often those most reluctant to speak out in support of the Code and often those who promote the products.

So persuasive is the practice of doctors accepting "gifts" from the pharmaceutical companies that a 1991 study published in *Pediatrics* found that the pharmaceutical industry spends $6,000–$8,000 in promotion *per doctor per year*. Expenditures for these special events increased fourteen-fold between 1975 and 1988. In Great Britain, it was found that thirty-one of the government's fifty-nine advisors on health and nutrition policy admitted to receiving payments from the food and drug industries, including the baby milk companies.

Doctors assure patients that these gifts do not influence them, but a 1994 study shows otherwise. Drs. Chren and Ladefeld examined the interactions with drug companies of forty "case" physicians, who had recommended specific drugs be added to an institution's list of approved drugs, and compared them with eighty "control" physicians. The results were published in the *Journal of the American Medical Association*. The authors found that by giving physicians money, the companies are successful in influencing doctors to recommend their products.

Can what applies to individuals be different for organizations? A 1986 internal memo from the AAP (obtained by *The Wall Street Journal*) stated that the Academy's Executive Committee "agreed that there is a need to make this statement [about marketing formula through pediatricians rather than directly to the consumer] reaffirming the AAP's position on marketing, breastmilk, lay advertising, etc. If there is a marketing war, there may be a shift in industry's distribution of funds and the AAP may have to cut back on anticipated income from the industry."

This financial coziness is showing some signs of strain. At the International Congress on Nutrition in Adelaide, Australia, in 1993, protests that the Congress was taking funds from three formula companies were ignored by the organizers, so a candlelight vigil was organized. Over 450 signatures were gathered in a petition that simply stated that the decision to accept infant formula industry support to the International Congress on Nutrition was wrong and recommended future Congresses not receive support from manufacturers of infant formula. Lung conferences are not supported by the tobacco industry because of conflict of interest, and the same should hold true for formula companies and infant feeding.

Other groups seem to have heard the message. The Canadian Pediatric Society has announced that it will no longer promote industry-sponsored parties at the society's annual meeting. The World Organization of Family Physicians and the International Midwifery Conference barred formula makers from their gatherings in British Columbia. Across the ocean, the Indian Academy of Paediatric and Conference Organizers recently refused to accept a donation from one infant formula company that was enough to fund their entire conference (estimated to be in excess of $250,000).

IBFAN has drafted a statement on baby milk companies' sponsorship of conferences that deal with infant feeding, stating that any conference or meeting that deals with infant or young child health or nutrition should not be financially sponsored by companies that produce or market products meant for infant or young child feeding. Perhaps the fact that these issues are being addressed more openly will continue discouraging professionals from accepting such commercial support.

THE DISCHARGE DEBATE

The discharge pack is another area where formula companies hope to both appear benevolent and gain valuable market share. Discharge or starter packs are "gift" packages filled with bottles, nipples, rattles, formula, pamphlets, and coupons given—free of charge—to new mothers when they leave the hospital with their newborns. This is an extremely important contact with potential consumers, as research has shown that 93% of mothers will continue to buy the brand of formula given to them at the hospital.

While the packs appear to be small, insignificant gifts, they are a key marketing strategy. The role of the starter pack is neither small nor insignificant. Indeed, companies make major contributions to hospitals to ensure their products are distributed. In 1989, Abbott Laboratories offered $500,000 to the Grace Hospital in Vancouver, Canada, in a bidding war with Bristol Myers for the privilege of "donating" formula supplies over three years. At this hospital, Canada's largest birthing facility, 85% of maternity patients express a desire to breastfeed, yet by the second day of life, 75% of infants are either given glucose water or formula. Such supplementation sabotages the breastfeeding relationship and sets the stage for insufficient milk syndrome. The availability and promotion of alternative foods has a demoralizing influence on both individual and social confidence in breastfeeding.

Mead Johnson has signed contracts to pay two Canadian hospitals for the right to give away free supplies of baby formula. The contract called for the Woman's College Hospital in Toronto to receive $1 million, plus $35,000 per year, to use only Mead Johnson baby formula for ten years and for the Royal Columbian Hospital in British Columbia to receive the same amount for a five-year deal. At the Isaac Killam Hospital in Halifax, Ross Laboratories paid $1 million in exchange for an exclusive contract to provide samples of its products to new mothers.

Ross Laboratories also proposed to pay The Doctor's Hospital in Canada $1 million for the privilege of providing all supplies of infant formula. Action for Corporate Accountability published the key points of the company proposal (provided by INFACT, Canada). It specified the hospital would:

- have access to Ross's architectural services for nurseries (when companies that sell infant formula provide free architectural design, nurseries and maternity wards are generally placed at great distances from each other, thus encouraging use of bottle-feeding)
- be *required* to provide Take Home packs to *all* new mothers, both breastfeeding and formula-feeding moms
- be supplied with Ross videos for breastfeeding mothers. These are the same videotapes sent to pregnant women in the United States who have made their intent to breastfeed known to their doctors or in their childbirth classes. Not only do the videos contain flawed information and images of breastfeeding and subliminal messages promoting the convenience of bottle-feeding, they also include within the jacket of the video box samples of formula and coupons to buy more formula.

Clearly, the discharge packs are anything but benign. Practically every U.S. hospital that provides maternity services now gives starter packs to mothers. The packages not only encourage women to formula-feed, they also encourage women to abandon breastfeeding sooner. In one study of breastfeeding low-income mothers published in *Pediatrics*, one group of women received a breastfeeding pack—containing breastfeeding pamphlets and breast pads—at hospital discharge, while the other group received a standard starter pack—including bottles, nipples, sterilized water, and pamphlets, but no formula. The group that received the standard pack began using formula for weekly feedings much sooner than the group that received the breastfeeding pack. The researchers concluded that the packs send subtle messages of "here's a set-up for formula for when you need it." This serves to make mothers feel insecure about the value of breastmilk and the feasibility of breastfeeding.

THE "BABY-FRIENDLY" EFFORT IS LAUNCHED

Health officials have long been concerned that hospitals should be places where breastfeeding is promoted. In 1991, UNICEF and WHO launched a worldwide Baby Friendly Hospital Initiative (BFHI) in a global effort to encourage and recognize hospitals that have implemented optimal lactation management. By implementing "Baby-Friendly" policies, hospitals can give breastfeeding mothers the information, confidence, and skills needed to initiate and continue breastfeeding. The program began with twelve "starter" countries, which included Turkey, Mexico, and Pakistan, before going worldwide in 1992 to empower women to breastfeed and to end the supply of free and low-cost infant formula. The first countries to adopt the Baby-Friendly guidelines were the Ivory Coast and Gabon, two French-speaking nations.

The BFHI is designed to remove hospital barriers to breastfeeding and to create an environment in which mothers can breastfeed in an informed and supportive setting. The basis of the BFHI is "Ten Steps to Successful Breastfeeding," a set of guidelines for hospitals, that ensures all mothers have accurate information on the benefits and techniques of breastfeeding (Table 5.4).

For a hospital to participate in the "Baby-Friendly Hospital Initiative" it must first sign a Certificate of Intent. The staff then receive training and relevant educational materials. After the training, if the hospital implements the "Ten Steps to Successful Breastfeeding" it is accredited as "Baby-Friendly." But this alone is not enough. Figure 5.8 shows the four key elements essential for effective breastfeeding programs.

Getting rid of the bottles, nipples, pacifiers, formula, and sterilized water is an important step. But another big obstacle in the quest to be baby friendly is the routine separation of mothers from their babies. It is common practice in many hospitals to keep the babies together in the nursery and the mothers in the wards. Some hospitals even have the nursery on a different floor than the mothers. Rooming-in greatly facilitates the establishment of breastfeeding.

At the end of its first full year, BFHI had achieved many gains. More than 700 hospitals around the world were close to becoming, or had been designated, "Baby Friendly." Asian countries have led the world in transforming hospitals to baby-friendliness. Recent counts include 102 Baby-Friendly hospitals in the Philippines, 97 in Indonesia, 45 in Thailand, and 21 in China. Many Latin American countries are working on legislation to encompass the entire International Code of Marketing of Breastmilk Substitutes; Brazil adopted such a law in 1992. Kenya has also adopted a model law to protect breastfeeding and to control marketing practices.

In the United States there is no comprehensive national program that fo-

Table 5.4
Becoming Baby Friendly: Ten Steps to Successful Breastfeeding

Each facility providing maternity services and care
for newborn infants should:

1. have a written breastfeeding policy that is routinely communicated to all health care staff

2. train all health care staff in skills necessary to implement this policy

3. inform all pregnant women about the benefits and management of breastfeeding

4. help mothers initiate breastfeeding within a half-hour of birth

5. show mothers how to breastfeed and how to maintain lactation even if they should be separated from their infants

6. give newborn infants no food or drink other than breastmilk, unless *medically* indicated

7. practice rooming-in—allow mothers and infants to remain together—twenty-four hours a day

8. encourage breastfeeding on demand

9. give no artificial teats or pacifiers (also called dummies or soothers) to breastfeeding infants

10. foster the establishment of breastfeeding support groups and refer mothers to them on discharge from the hospital or clinic

cuses on breastfeeding promotion. The U.S. Department of Health and Human Services recently funded a $500,000 feasibility study to see what adaptations would be required to achieve baby-friendly success in the United States. In June 1994, the Healthy Mothers, Healthy Babies coalition, which conducted the study, issued a report. Both the study and the report have been highly controversial. Critics have charged that breastfeeding activists were excluded from participating and that the baby milk industry determined the outcome of the report before the study was even undertaken.

In the meantime, some U.S. hospitals are preparing themselves for Baby-Friendly status in order to be ready to receive certification once the recommendations come out. To date, 143 hospitals and 3 birthing centers, representing 36 states and the District of Columbia, have received certificates of intent. Unfortunately, many U.S. hospitals are privately owned and any initiative coming from the department of Health and Human Services can be ignored. Efforts continue, but two additional facets of the current U.S. health care system pose obstacles to the baby-friendly movement: liability concerns and early discharge.

The BFHI is a serious attempt to use hospitals for promoting breastfeed-

Figure 5.8
Four Key Elements of Breastfeeding Programs

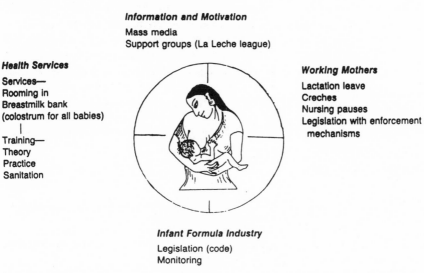

Information and Motivation
Mass media
Support groups (La Leche league)

Health Services

Services—
Rooming in
Breastmilk bank
(colostrum for all babies)
|
Training—
Theory
Practice
Sanitation

Working Mothers
Lactation leave
Creches
Nursing pauses
Legislation with enforcement
    mechanisms

Infant Formula Industry
Legislation (code)
Monitoring

Source: N. Baumslag, *Mother and Child Health: Delivering the Services* (Oxford: Oxford University Press, 1994).

ing, rather than using them for undermining breastfeeding. However, using the hospital setting for promoting breastfeeding can only be effective when the mothers actually stay in the hospital until they are able to breastfeed to their and the staff's satisfaction. In many hospitals around the world, women typically stayed from 3 to 7 days following a normal delivery. However, the length of stay worldwide is being shortened. In the United States, the length of the hospital stay has been decreasing as insurance companies limit the amount of time they will pay for a new mother to reside in the hospital following delivery. Insurance companies are now dictating that women stay no more than two nights following a vaginal (or uncomplicated) birth. Some insurers only permit a one night stay, while others provide a large cash bonus to the mother if she leaves voluntarily after one night. Typically, hospital rooms are counted at midnight, so that a woman who delivers her baby late in the evening on a Wednesday and is approved for a one night stay must check out of the hospital Thursday morning. In an environment where the role of the hospital is to deliver the baby, and not a place to recover, it is very hard to provide education and guidance. The woman who checks out the morning after her delivery has not had time to attend new baby classes, meet with a lactation consultant, or practice breastfeeding in the presence of a skilled nurse. It doesn't need to be this way. At the José Favella Hospital in the Philippines, mothers are not discharged until they have demonstrated their ability to breastfeed.

The most important tenet of the "baby-friendly" initiative is that babies stay with mothers, ending the practice of routine separation of mother and child. But the insurance companies don't want the babies to stay with the mother. From a liability point of view, it is much safer for all the babies to be in a locked room under the charge of nurses. Having babies all over the maternity floor raises fears in hospital staff and insurance companies that women will drop their babies or the babies will be kidnapped—and that the hospital will be sued. Concerns over security and potential legal action need to be considered, but should not outweigh the compelling need for mother and child to be together.

THE WIC PROGRAM

In 1974, the Federal Government established the Special Supplemental Food Program for Women, Infants and Children (called the WIC program) in an attempt to lower the strikingly high U.S. rates of infant mortality and morbidity. WIC serves poor women and children who are at the greatest nutritional risk. Participants in WIC receive food vouchers for eggs, cheese, cereal, juice, milk, and infant formula. WIC is made available to selected pregnant, postpartum, and breastfeeding women, as well as to children up to five. When WIC began in 1974, it served 88,000 participants, of whom 26,000 were infants. In 1994 it served 6.5 million and 1.8 million were infants. The WIC food costs were $8.2 million in 1974 and $2,335 million in 1994.

Even though WIC is extremely effective, funding limitations restrict WIC from serving up to 50% of mothers who meet its eligibility requirements. Increases in unemployment, Medicaid referrals, and the overall awareness of the program have led to a steady increase in applicants. Not only does WIC serve fewer participants than qualify, but it doesn't serve those it does fully. WIC supplies formula-feeding mothers with only two-thirds of the formula needed to nourish an infant properly. The difference can either be made up by the mother purchasing additional formula or by simply diluting what she does have. Diluting robs the child of essential nutrition and leads to health problems. In order to save money, many mothers purchase whatever brand of formula that is on sale, switching brands of formula routinely, or adding cereals early, which also leads to medical problems.

A primary reason why WIC is so limited in how fully it serves and in how many people it *can* serve is the large share of its budget that is used for purchasing infant formula. Hundreds of millions of dollars each year go to purchasing formula that will then be given away to program participants. The current figure of $523 million spent on formula represents 28% of the program's total annual food costs and amounts to almost $25 per month, per infant. Yet, even at its current funding levels, *WIC provides free formula to 37% of all babies born in the United States each year.*

WIC mothers are far less likely to breastfeed than other American women, even though the very children WIC aims to serve—those living in poverty with little access to health care—are those who would most benefit from the immunological and nutritional properties of breastmilk. And since Medicaid pays the health costs of most WIC infants, taxpayers are, in fact, paying not only for infant formula but also for the child's higher rate of medical problems.

WIC began taking breastfeeding promotion seriously in 1989 when each state agency was required to hire a state nursing coordinator, write a plan to promote breastfeeding, and ensure adequate breastfeeding support for mothers. State agencies were given a total of $8 million per year for that purpose, which translated into $10 per pregnant and lactating client. As a result, 12% more of its clients are now breastfeeding (though not necessarily exclusively). However, the $8 million has remained fixed for five years, during which time the WIC population has nearly doubled. Breastfeeding advocates have worked to raise that allotment to $21 per pregnant and lactating woman for breastfeeding education and support (as opposed to having a maximum dollar amount) when WIC funds are appropriated.

Breastfeeding advocates are also trying to see that a standard method for the states to track breastfeeding participants is established. Until recently, the United States did not track breastfeeding patterns but instead relied on statistics collected by Abbott Laboratories, makers of Similac (the most successful brand of formula in the country)—statistics that have been used in the planning and budgeting of federal programs. Efforts are underway for WIC to collect these statistics. The definition of breastfeeding also has to be addressed because the current definition—breastfeeding at least once a day—grossly exaggerates the number of infants actually breastfeeding and does not indicate the number of infants being exclusively breastfed.

The value of breastmilk is as compelling economically as it is nutritionally and immunologically. If every WIC participant today decided to breastfeed, it would save over $500 million a year in federal funds—and that doesn't take into account that the children would be healthier, translating into significant indirect savings.

No examination of how best to help our nation's poor women and at-risk babies is complete without looking at the larger issue of infant feeding and, specifically, the lack of breastfeeding. When WIC participants breastfeed, the mothers provide the best nourishment and their babies receive the best food source and the maximum protection against allergies and disease. Taxpayers save millions. And with the millions of dollars saved, WIC could open its arms to the needy families that it now turns away.

SUPPLYING WIC WITH FORMULA

The infant formula companies routinely bid against each other for the opportunity to supply the WIC program's formula needs. After years of suspect bids, the pricing practices of infant formula companies came under scrutiny. Allegations of collusion, unfair pricing, and monopoly behavior were asserted amid complaints of frequent, substantial, and parallel price increases by Abbott Laboratories (Similac), Bristol Myers (Enfamil), and American Home Products (SMA). These three formula manufacturers dominate the infant formula market (the first two ring up more than 90% of U.S. formula sales).

Each of these three companies raised their prices a dozen times during the 1980s and early 1990s. Between 1980 and 1987, the cost of formula doubled and was six times more expensive than cow's milk (its primary ingredient). The U.S. Senate, the House of Representatives, and the Federal Trade Commission initiated antitrust investigations due to overpricing by formula companies. Senator Metzenbaum brought this issue to the public with hearings in May 1990 before the Senate Judiciary Committee on Antitrust, Monopolies, and Business Rights. The Federal Trade Commission followed with an investigation in September 1992 to examine the complaints of unfair pricing. The Florida Attorney General, along with twenty-seven food and drug store chains, sued the three major formula companies, alleging that they conspired to rig bids, drive up prices, and keep other firms out of the industry. In addition, nine states have since instigated lawsuits for alleged price fixing.

These price rises were particularly onerous to the WIC program because, as noted before, WIC received a fixed amount each year; any increase in formula price translated directly into a decrease in the number of program participants. As formula prices went up, hundreds of thousands of women and children were eliminated from the program at a time when the number of poor households was on the rise.

Poor mothers who could not participate in WIC were forced to spend more of their scant resources on formula, work longer hours in order to pay for formula, or "stretch" formula by overdiluting it, causing diarrhea and marasmus (starvation wasting). Budget cuts and recessionary times are usually blamed for the fact that WIC cannot serve its entire target population, but the real reason WIC is unable to serve more eligible participants is because so much of the money ear-marked to help people is funneled into the coffers of the formula companies.

Bristol Myers and American Home Products settled their federal antitrust case in the fall of 1992 and Abbott Laboratories settled its case in the spring of 1993. In all, the three companies agreed to pay $250 million in settlements (an amount, according to *American Lawyer*, equaling less than a year's pretax profits for Ross Laboratories), but have denied any wrong-doing. The settlement ends a major legal action without resolving any issues of guilt. There is nothing to stop the companies from continuing to set prices just as they have in the past. Nor will consumers benefit from the $250 million settlement. Only direct purchasers (such as "Toys R Us" and supermarket chains) can recover monies as a result of the antitrust actions. An Abbott spokesperson said they were pleased to have the matter settled and noted that the settlement would not have an impact on net earnings.

The status quo remains. Formula companies continue to produce artificial milks at great profit. Women continue to choose formula over breast-feeding. And the government continues to pick up the tab, both for the formula and the formula-related illnesses. The antitrust action sought to curb abuses by the industry, but it is not clear that the abuses or the profit motive have been curbed at all. In the meantime, taxpayers continue to subsidize the formula companies.

HOW SHOULD FORMULA BE SOLD?

In industrialized nations, infant formula manufacturers have long marketed their products through physicians rather than going directly to the consumer. Operating under the guidelines of an industry-approved anti-advertising code, products have been promoted by pharmaceutical companies through an extensive, and carefully cultivated, network of doctor and hospital relationships. This medical sales method is known as "ethical marketing." The stated reasons for selling this way are that physicians can best apprise a mother of her baby's nutritional needs and that breastfeeding is so important as to outweigh any restrictions on competition.

In the mid-1980s, Nestlé decided to tackle the American market for infant formula, where it had almost no presence. As a food company, it was not well positioned to penetrate into hospitals and medical offices. It decided to launch two new brands, Good Start and Good Nature brands of "follow-up formula," directly to the consumer. In addition, they ignored the anti-advertising standard and began an extensive television and magazine advertising campaign.

In 1993, Nestlé Food Company filed a lawsuit against the leading American producers of baby formula and the American Academy of Pediatrics (AAP), alleging a conspiracy to block competitors from the lucrative U.S. market. The suit alleged that Abbott Laboratories and Bristol Myers conspired with the AAP to create a Code of Marketing Practices that discouraged direct advertising of baby formula. Nestlé contended that the large sales force required under the system of "ethical marketing" is an artificial barrier to the market and violates anti-trust law. Bolstering their case is Federal Trade Commission (FTC) testimony before Congress concerning the formula industry. Mary Lou Steptoe, the FTC's Deputy Director of Competition, stated, "The anti-trust laws do prohibit agreements among competitors to refrain from advertising, even where the competitors profess laudatory motives such as the public health or safety." Additionally, the Justice Department told the industry their anti-advertising code might well violate anti-trust laws.

It is hard to know who's most to blame for the latest of corporate wars or their strategies. Is it better to have greedy companies, colluding with doctors, marketing essentially identical products through people who gain by recommending them? Or is it better to open the floodgates to competition and let the free market determine the victors? In either scenario, the consumers are the clear losers. Breastmilk substitutes can be useful, life-saving products; no one suggests they should not exist for the times where need may arise. But just because they can save lives under very specific circumstances, it does not mean that they should be widely distributed and vigorously promoted. Insulin, for example, can save the lives of diabetics, but no good doctor would ever advocate the use of insulin unless it were strictly necessary. One approach to take might be to put formula in the same category as insulin and make it fall under a drug classification available only by prescription.

The Director General of Pakistan's Ministry of Health announced that infant formula and baby foods would be placed on a pharmaceutical list because infant mortality and diarrheal deaths were so high and bottle-feeding so rampant. The plan was to ban advertising of the products and restrict availability to prescription status only. Nestlé Infant Foods Manager, Geoffrey Fookes, flew to Islamabad to protest the decision, and somehow the Director General was persuaded to halt this plan.

Papua New Guinea did succeed in limiting access to artificial foods. Aware that plastic bottles were a major source of germs, legislation was passed in 1977 to control the use of feeding bottles and artificial milk. It was made illegal to sell a bottle without a prescription and a health worker had to prove it was in a baby's interests to be bottle-fed before writing a prescription. What happened? Malnutrition was reduced noticeably. In 1976, a third of children under two in the capital, Port Moresby, were being artificially fed, and over two-thirds of these were malnourished. In just three years, bottle-feeding had dropped to 12%, and malnutrition had been reduced by a third. There is a higher level of awareness of the barriers to breastfeeding and the value of breastfeeding as part of total health care among health workers. Papua New Guinea, where 85% of the population lives in rural areas and only 10% have access to safe drinking water, had an infant mortality rate comparable in 1985 with Brazil and lower than that of South Africa, Turkey, and Saudi Arabia—all countries considered to be at a more "advanced" level of development.

Another approach to the dilemma of how to limit bottle-feeding is to tax formula, either with a luxury tax (snack foods and high-ticket items are often subject to a higher sales tax) or a sin tax (as tobacco and alcohol products are taxed). In either case, revenues from the extra tax dollars could be directed to programs that help infants. On the other hand, any tax that increased the price of formula could result in increased infant malnutrition and death. Providing a tax relief rather than a tax burden might be a better strategy. The U.S. Department of Agriculture is considering recommending tax relief to mothers who breastfeed for four to six months as part of a series of steps designed to produce substantial health gains and to lead to improvements in both the quality and quantity of life.

Discussions about whether formula should be taxed, whether the industry should be able to advertise, whether formula should be classified as a drug instead of food, and whether the use of the product causes unnecessary deaths bring to mind a different debate this country has been waging for decades: how tobacco products should be advertised and distributed. In both instances, the debate involves public health versus private profit. There are numerous similarities between the infant formula industry and the tobacco industry, and there are many ways in which formula and cigarettes are similar, but the main point is that as medical researchers reveal the damage caused by these products, public attitudes have shifted. Public policy and societal acceptance of these products only change as attitudes and priorities shift. Perhaps the change in nonacceptance of smoking, especially in public, and the increased efforts to regulate tobacco products should be seen as a hopeful sign that the tide can turn against the notion that bottle-feeding formula is "normal" and as healthy as breastfeeding.

WHERE ARE WE NOW?

The world has clearly navigated the turn back towards breastfeeding. (James Grant, UNICEF Executive Director, 1994)

The early 1990s has seen a leap in breastfeeding promotion activities for governments all through the world. Nations have reaffirmed the importance and benefits of breastfeeding to infants, mothers, and society at large in four key documents published by UNICEF/WHO: *The Innocenti Declaration on the Protection, Promotion and Support of Breastfeeding* (Table 5.5), *The Convention on the Rights of The Child, The Declaration of the World Summit on Children,* and *The World Declaration on Nutrition and Plan of Action for Nutrition.*

Recognizing the need to protect, support, and promote breastfeeding and to monitor formula company violations of the Code, in 1992 seventeen organizations formed the World Alliance for Breastfeeding Action (WABA) and launched the first annual World Breastfeeding Week. The first week of

Table 5.5

The Innocenti Declaration on the Protection, Promotion and Support of Breastfeeding

---

RECOGNIZING that

Breastfeeding is a unique process that:

- provides ideal nutrition for infants and contributes to their healthy growth and development;

- reduces incidence and severity of infectious diseases, thereby lowering infant morbidity and mortality;

- contributes to women's health by reducing the risks of breast and ovarian cancer, and by increasing the spacing between pregnancies;

- provides social and economic benefits to the family and the nation;

- provides most women with a sense of satisfaction when successfully carried out; and

Recent research has found that:

- these benefits increase with increased exclusiveness of breastfeeding during the first six months of life and thereafter with increased duration of breastfeeding with complementary foods, and

- programme interventions can result in positive changes in breastfeeding behaviour;

WE THEREFORE DECLARE that

As a global goal for optimal maternal and child health and nutrition, all women should be enabled to practise exclusive breastfeeding and all infants should be fed exclusively on breast milk from 4–6 months of age. Thereafter, children should continue to be breastfed, while receiving appropriate and adequate complementary foods, for up to two years of age or beyond. This child-feeding ideal is to be achieved by creating an appropriate environment of awareness and support so that women can breastfeed in this manner.

Source: WHO/UNICEF, *Innocenti Declaration on the Protection, Promotion and Support of Breastfeeding*, produced and adopted at the WHO/UNICEF policymakers' meeting on "Breastfeeding in 1990s: A Global Initiative," co-sponsored by the U.S. Agency for International Development (USAID) and the Swedish International Development Authority (SIDA), Spedale degli Innocenti, Florence, Italy, July 30–August 1, 1990.

each August, people worldwide join together in celebration in support of breastfeeding. In addition, the WHO/UNICEF Baby-Friendly Hospital Initiative is changing the breastfeeding climate in hospitals around the world. As part of this effort, UNICEF's Executive Director, James Grant, has urged physicians the world over to make a pledge to "protect, promote and support breastfeeding and to work to end the free and low-cost distribution of breastmilk substitutes in our health care systems" (Appendix F). Many groups are working on different fronts using a variety of strategies to in-

Figure 5.9
Breastfeeding Promotion

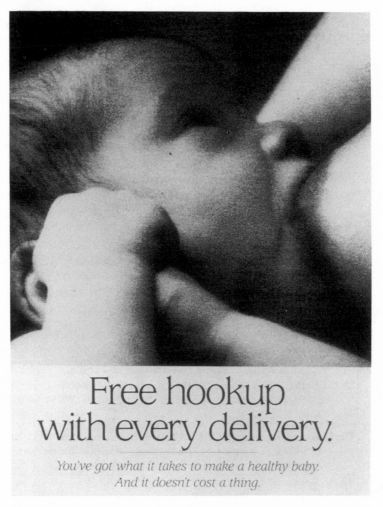

Free hookup
with every delivery.

You've got what it takes to make a healthy baby.
And it doesn't cost a thing.

This poster was one of many displayed throughout Canada as part of a breastfeeding awareness campaign. *Photo courtesy*: INFACT, Canada.

crease breastfeeding awareness and to raise breastfeeding rates. One example of this is the series of posters, displayed in public places and designed to develop more public awareness of breastfeeding, created by the Canadian group of INFACT (Figure 5.9).

The activities of the past several decades have been difficult and frequently tragic. Health professionals and ordinary citizens alike have ex-

Table 5.6
A Half-Century Movement to Limit Inappropriate Use of Breastmilk Supplies

1939	Cicely Williams's speech *Milk and Murder* recommends that deaths resulting from misguided propaganda on infant feeding should be "regarded as murder."
1968	Dr. Derrick Jelliffe coins the term "commerciogenic malnutrition" to describe the impact of marketing practices on infant health.
1974	The World Health Assembly recommends regulating inappropriate sales promotion of infant foods used to replace breastmilk.
1977	Nestlé boycott is launched to protest marketing practices.
1979	WHO/UNICEF host international meeting on infant and young child.
1981	International Code of Marketing of Breastmilk Substitutes adopted at World Health Assembly, with United States casting the sole vote of opposition.
1984	The Nestlé boycott ends.
1986	World Health Assembly passes resolution banning free and subsidized supplies.
1988	The Nestlé boycott is restarted and broadened to include American Home Products.
1990	The *Innocenti Declaration* calls upon all governments to enact the Ten Steps to Successful Breastfeeding and the International Code.
1991	UNICEF and WHO launch the Baby-Friendly Hospital Initiative in sixteen starter countries. UNICEF calls for end of all free supplies. Formula manufacturers promise to end supplies in developing countries by 1992.
1992	UNICEF and WHO expand BFHI to a worldwide movement. Hundreds of thousands of women participate in the first annual "World Breastfeeding Week."
1994	The United States reverses its opposition to the International Marketing Code. The Code is adopted by international consensus at the World Health Assembly.
2000	????

pended tremendous time and used limited resources in a continuing battle to get the infant formula industry to be held accountable. Lives have been lost and scarce resources squandered (Figure 5.10). Each time it has seemed the tide was turned, industry has developed new strategies with its might.

Even today, over 4,000 babies worldwide die every day because they are not breastfed. In poor societies, bottle-fed babies are up to twenty-five times more likely to die. But the problem is not just one affecting babies in far-away, impoverished lands. A baby in a wealthy country who is bottle-fed is five times more likely to contract gastroenteritis than a breastfed one—

**Figure 5.10
Wasting Resources**

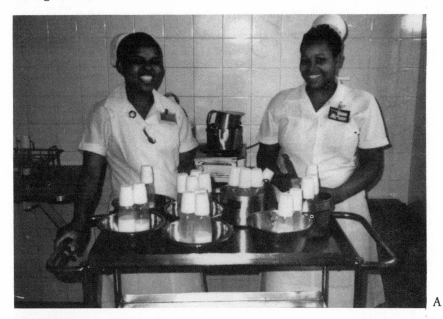

A

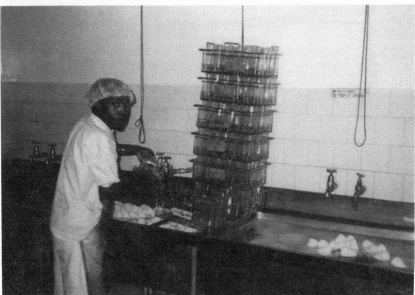

B

Using artificial foods requires extra staff, as seen in these photos from South Africa: (A) Two full-time, trained staff nurses spent their day mixing Lactogen for pediatric patients; (B) A full-time employee was required just to wash infant feeding bottles. South Africa now has a very progressive breastfeeding policy. *Photo courtesy*: N. Baumslag.

regardless of socio-economic conditions. For every 1,000 infants born in the United States each year, four will die because they are not breastfed.

UNICEF had asked Nestlé to end bottle-feeding promotion, including free supplies, in all countries by the end of 1994, regardless of government action. Nestlé has failed to name a single country where it has stopped free supplies. Not only has Nestlé broken agreements to curtail free milk, it has also lobbied to weaken government legislation and increased its promotional activities. Using calculated high visibility strategies to portray itself as a benevolent institution, Nestlé circles the globe looking for good deeds to perform. In Canada recently, Nestlé was the official corporate sponsor of "National Year of the Family."

The struggle to make breastfeeding the norm once again has been long and slow (Table 5.6). Who knows how long the boycott will last this time and how much time, energy, and money will be spent fighting the same battles that have been waged for decades? Despite the unequal battle for the breast of might against right, there is some good news. Breastfeeding awareness has increased. More and more, women are breastfeeding their infants. At many levels, we are seeing the reintroduction of a breastfeeding culture with a vigorous defense despite incursions of a bottle-feeding culture. The battle is still raging, but the sense of change is stronger than it has ever been.

Six

Women and Work

Breast-feeding is . . . a communion between mother and child that, like marriage, is "intimate to the degree of being sacred." . . . We conclude that the Constitution protects from excessive state interference a woman's decision respecting breast-feeding her child.
—Judgment from U.S. Appeals Court, 1981

More and more women are entering the formal work force. Formerly, in nonindustrial societies, women breastfed until the onset of, or the preparation for, the next pregnancy. This provided the women with a natural form of birth control (see "The Breasts and Contraception" in chapter 3) and provided the child with a steady flow of nature's bounty. However, this has changed as increasing numbers of women have moved into urban, industrial centers. Increasingly, working women now breastfeed only until the time they resume employment outside the home.

In societies where women stay home with the baby for a year, most mothers breastfeed for a year. In societies where women stay home with the baby for four months, most mothers breastfeed for four months. In societies where women stay home with the baby for six weeks, most mothers breastfeed for six weeks. In the United States, only 13% of the women who return to work full-time shortly after giving birth breastfeed for at least six months, significantly fewer than those who stay home. And women who attempt to combine breastfeeding and work often find the barriers in the workplace insurmountable.

No longer does the length of time breastfeeding correspond to the spacing between children. The length of breastfeeding now corresponds largely with the spacing between the birth and the return to employment. It is ironic that this is so, because it is entirely possible to combine working and

Table 6.1
Key Benefits of Breastfeeding

TO NATION	TO EMPLOYER[*]	TO EMPLOYEE	TO CHILD
Release of scarce medical funds and staff	Increased productivity and company loyalty	Closer bond with child	Closer bond with mother
Savings of foreign exchange	Greater employee satisfaction	Saves money	Gets sick less often and illnesses are less severe
Less environmental waste and pollution	Lower absentee rate	Convenient, clean, and prewarmed	Lower incidence of sudden infant death syndrome
Less demand for agricultural and energy resources	Lower turnover among workers/ reduced training costs	Contraceptive benefit	Greater protection against allergies, asthma, and diabetes
	Fewer demands on employee health benefits	Faster recovery from birth	Greater protection against communicable and infectious diseases
		Protection against breast, cervical, and ovarian cancers	Provides optimal growth and neurological development
		Lower rate of urinary tract infections	Higher IQ
		Reduces the risk of hip fractures and osteoporosis	Less dental decay
		Greater satisfaction in job/income security	Less heart disease and cancer in later life

*If nursing breaks and daycare provisions are provided

breastfeeding—but the perception is that the two must be exclusive. "Women and Work" is a significant subject, and the issues that affect women in the workplace are issues that we must all face if we are concerned with infant and maternal health. The battle for the breast has been largely waged around limiting the grasp of formula marketers. But as we approach the year 2000, the battle will be lost unless there is recognition of the importance of breastfeeding to everyone in society (Table 6.1) and women are given the opportunity to breastfeed.

THE WORK OF WOMEN

Images of women come and go like the tide. "You've come a long way, baby" was the slogan of the 70s that came to symbolize the strides women had made in gaining equality. The 80s hero was Superwoman—she had a successful career, a stable marriage, was a loving mother to 2.5 perfect children, had a spotlessly clean house, was a gourmet cook, spoke three languages, and taught aerobics on weekends after reaching multiple orgasms. But this notion of a modern day Superwoman faded by the end of the 80s as the image collided with the realities and stresses of everyday life. The 90s woman is more complex: she may be recently divorced, or in a second marriage; she may have children and/or stepchildren who commute between parents with a dizzying schedule based on shared custody; she may work part-time or in the informal sector, without any workplace benefits, or she may have a challenging profession, but responsibilities for young children and aging parents add to her workload and stress level.

The complexity of the past several decades of social change has ushered in an entirely different picture of life than that seen in *Leave it to Beaver*. In most industrialized countries, the traditional family with the male as wage earner and the female as at-home mother has gone by the wayside. In the United States, only 11% of all married couples fit such a mold. In fact, the composition of the American family has changed in several ways. First, more U.S. women with children are working outside the home than ever before. In the United States, between 1950 and 1985, female participation in the labor force increased by 178% while the number of men in the work force rose by only 47%. Today, women make up 45% of the work force and by the year 2005 are expected to make up 47%. Eighty percent of women in the labor force are of childbearing age, and 93% of these women will become pregnant during their working lives. Fifty-eight percent of all mothers with pre-schoolers work outside the home, up from 34% in 1977. Twenty-five percent of all women workers hold part-time jobs; two-thirds of all part-time workers in 1992 were women.

Second, more men, when they are present in the home, are participating in ways their fathers never dreamed of. No longer content to be the vacant breadwinner, men are attending childbirth classes, assisting in labor and delivery, are more involved with their kids, and are even doing some housework. Third, female-headed households are increasing. High rates of divorce and record numbers of unwed mothers have launched the United States to first place in the developed world for single-parent households. It is estimated that 8.7 million women are raising 16 million children without husbands present in the home.

Women work harder than men whether they are eastern or western, housewives or job holders. A Pakistani woman spends sixty-three hours a week on domestic work alone, while a western housewife, despite her modern appliances, works just six hours less. According to labor economist Nancy Barrett, there is no evidence that sweeping changes in the division of labor within households have coincided with women's increasing labor force participation. Just because a woman does full-time paid work doesn't mean that she does any less of the unpaid work. In fact, the husbands of employed women help out less than do husbands of housewives, 36 minutes each day compared to 75 minutes, respectively. At least the perception is not different from the reality—in the United States, 90% of wives and 85% of husbands say that the woman does all or almost all of the household chores. The result is that American women work almost twenty-two hours more each week than do their male counterparts.

Women are competing fully in the work force, postponing childbearing, and returning to their jobs soon after each child is born. Juggling the demands of a family against the demands of a career requires constant balancing. Combining the responsibilities of work and mothering is difficult and tiring in the best of circumstances. For those who do it without partners, emotional and physical limits are easily reached. It is clear that women are the key; women shape the present and the future. Mothers are the vital link to the improvement of child and family health.

The whole process of reproduction does not always cooperate with the demands of the present day workplace. Some women feel great throughout their pregnancies and are able to work right up to the day they deliver. For others, morning sickness can be debilitating and/or bed rest may be required. The birth itself can be very hard on a woman's body; giving birth to twins (which is occurring at record levels) and cesarean sections (which occur for more than one out of five births) are especially hard physically.

The initial period after the birth is crucial in developing a close maternal relationship and in setting good attitudes about being a family. Breastfeeding plays a major role in establishing this relationship. In order for breastfeeding to succeed, there must be a positive societal attitude toward it coupled with the opportunity for the mother to spend enough time with the child to accomplish it. Breastfed babies are healthier, better protected from disease, and have a closer and more secure attachment to their mothers than babies who are formula fed.

Concerns about keeping a job and loss of income from extra leave affect almost every pregnancy. Employment cannot be combined with maternity unless the workplace can accommodate the various needs of women, including those needs that cannot be foreseen. This would be a fine theoretical issue were it not for the fact that at least 33% of the *entire* American labor force will become pregnant during their working lives. Given the compelling size of this issue, it is striking that, even today, the vast majority of American women have neither income nor job protection at the time of the birth. Women, more often than not, return to work sooner than they prefer due to financial stress and the fear of losing their jobs.

Workers need the security of knowing that caring for their families and themselves will not jeopardize their economic well-being. Women who breastfeed have healthier babies and save money by using their own readily available, highly nutritious, immunologically packed, and ecologically sound food source. Women who nurse their children are themselves better protected against breast and ovarian cancer and have a close and secure attachment to their babies. Yet maternal employment is often cited as a major contributing factor for the decline in the duration of breastfeeding. In a society where almost half of the mothers with children under one year work outside the home, many women feel that breastfeeding and employment are incompatible, a notion often perpetuated by health workers.

In 1985, the United Nations called for all nations to recognize the unremunerated contributions of women by reflecting their value in national statistics. The market cost method assesses women's home services at $16,000 per year (in 1991 U.S. dollars) based on research by the Bureau of Economic Analysis. This value is comparable to the average salary of a kindergarten teacher, hotel clerk, receptionist, or security guard. Replacement cost figures are similar. Another measure is opportunity cost—or how much potential income a woman is losing by not working. This figure is used widely by lawyers for divorce proceedings.

In the United States, it is estimated that 25–40% of the gross domestic product (GDP) is the true contribution of unpaid household work. In 1993, U.S. GDP was $6,378 billion. Using the lower estimate, women's unpaid work amounts to over $1,594 billion each year. The percentage of GDP attributed to household work in third-world countries is even higher, yet most countries have been sluggish about, or even unwilling to, include women's unpaid work in their national statistics. The new South Africa has, however, just stipulated that this be done in its new constitution.

Improving the means for women to bear and breastfeed children in a world that requires most women to work (and offers the option to those who can choose to work) is the most sane approach to attacking potential problems of all sorts in the next, and future, generations.

A HISTORICAL PERSPECTIVE OF MATERNITY ENTITLEMENTS

Historically, a woman's role in society was to provide children and child care, to gather food and water, to prepare food, and to keep house. Traditionally, when mothers worked, the extended family provided child care. In many cultures, the grandparents of each generation raise the children, enabling the parents an opportunity to better the family financially. Even today, throughout Europe and Asia, more than half of all young children are taken care of by their grandmothers.

In the United States, however, families have disintegrated, adult children no longer live near their parents, and delayed reproduction has led to more infirm parents for the adult children just starting their own families (the baby-boom generation has been renamed "the sandwich generation"). The joint burdens of child care and wage-earning generally belong to parents living as an isolated nuclear family and, increasingly, to the women who head single-parent families (Figure 6.1).

While women in industrialized societies view childbirth as a routine, if dramatic, event where both mother and baby thrive soon after the delivery, in the nonindustrialized world the lives of women are dominated by the risk of death during childbirth—thirty to fifty times greater than the risk of death experienced by women in the United States. The bulk of children on this planet live in third-world countries, where 50% of those born will not live to attend a day of school. For these youngsters, breastfeeding is not a luxury, it is the passport to life.

Early in this century, the concepts of maternity leave and lactation breaks were discussed by nations all around the world as a means of protecting newborns and lowering the infant mortality rates. In 1919, the International Labour Organization (ILO) resolved that a woman should be allowed *paid* maternity leave for six weeks following a birth and should be allowed to nurse her child twice a day for half an hour during working hours. In 1952, these maternity "protections" were strengthened by making available paid nursing breaks during working hours. The United States is among the many countries that accepted these conventions, though it would not be obvious to any observer. In other countries, like South Africa, strong trade unions have achieved maternity and health rights for women.

Over three-fourths of the countries in the world conform to the ILO conventions and offer twelve weeks or more maternity leave. Over half provide nursing breaks in the workplace, and approximately three-quarters provide job security (Table 6.2). Job security and pay during leave facilitate breastfeeding at home.

The criteria for granting maternity leave varies considerably. In some countries, state (or provincial) governments rather than the federal (or central) government are responsible for labor relations. Regulations may only apply to government employees. Qualifications for eligibility may depend on employment history. Paid maternity leave comes in many forms: Argentina, Barbados, Brazil, Colombia, Cuba, Ecuador, Peru, Guatemala, Uruguay, Mexico, Jamaica, Nicaragua, and Panama, provide 100% of wages during maternity leave; Botswana guarantees only a minimum of 25% of wages; in Greece, the government provides a single lump-sum allowance for confinement expenses and additional entitlements up to the equivalent of normal earnings during maternity leave only for women with

Figure 6.1
Breastfeeding and Work

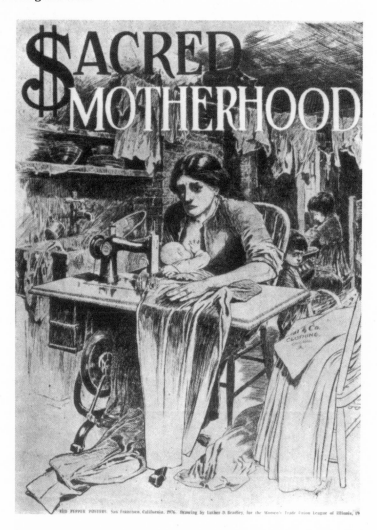

More women are working outside the home without any corresponding reduction in their home responsibilities. Here a garment
worker breastfeeds while she toils. *Source*: Bread and Roses.

social security coverage; Israel provides cash benefits and paid leave for
new mothers who have a hospital delivery, plus blanket and clothes for
the baby.

The United States is the only country in the world that does not provide for paid maternity leave. Of the many differences in everyday life

Table 6.2
A Survey of ILO Compliance

To successfully combine breastfeeding and working, a woman needs support in the workplace. Legislation is necessary to ensure that women receive adequate maternity leave and time during the day for breastfeeding and/or expressing milk. The following countries meet the first three International Labour Organization (ILO) standards.* Countries listed in bold type meet fourth standard as well:

ILO Standards

- 12 weeks maternity leave, with extension if necessary

- cash benefits during leave of at least 66% of previous earnings

- breastfeeding breaks totalling at least one hour per day

- prohibition of dismissal during maternity leave

Asia:

Fiji, **India, Iran, Israel, Mongolia**, Myanmar, New Zealand, Pakistan, **Sri Lanka**

The Americas:

Argentina, Bolivia, Brazil, Canada, **Chile, Colombia, Costa Rica,** Cuba, **Dominican Republic, Ecuador,** El Salvador, Grenada, **Guatemala, Haiti,** Jamaica, **Mexico, Nicaragua, Panama, Peru, Uruguay, Venezuela**

Africa:

Angola, **Benin, Burkina Faso, Cameroon, Congo, Egypt, Equatorial Africa, Gabon, Ghana,** Guinea, Ivory Coast, Liberia, **Libya, Nigeria, Senegal,** Togo, **Zaire, Zambia**

Europe:

Albania, Austria, Azerbaijan, Belgium, **Bosnia-Herzegovina, Bulgaria, Byelorussia, Czechoslovakian Republic,** Denmark, Finland, **France, Germany,** Greece, **Hungary,** Iceland, Ireland, **Italy, Kyrgyzstan, Luxemburg,** Malta, **Netherlands, Norway, Poland, Portugal, Romania, Russia,** Slovenia, Spain, Sweden, **Tajikistan, Turkey, Ukraine,** United Kingdom

*The Maternity Protection Convention (No. 3), 1919; and 1952 revision (No. 103).

Sources: The Clearinghouse on Infant/Maternal Nutrition, "Legislation and Policies to Support Maternal and Child Nutrition," No. 6, Washington, DC, 6/89, updated 5/93; International Labour Organization, "Protection of Working Mothers: An ILO Global Survey (1964-1984)," *Women at Work*, No. 2, Switzerland, 1984; The International Code Documentation Centre, Penang, Malaysia.

Table 6.3
European "Family Values"

What every mother gets	No. weeks paid maternity leave	% earnings	Comments
Belgium	14	80	
France	16	90	Unpaid job protection for two years
Germany	14	100	Supplementary benefits available for up to eighteen months
Italy	20	80	
Norway	18	100	Working mother can take one hour each day (two if in public sector) to breastfeed or pump
Portugal	12	100	
Sweden	78	100	Six-hour workday until child turns eight
United States	0	0	

that exist on the opposite sides of the Atlantic Ocean, none is greater than the differences in approach between Americans and Europeans. In Europe, the government is charged with providing expansive family benefit programs. Workers pay up to 44% of each paycheck in taxes to ensure a wide range of family-related services, protecting workers against three basic contingencies: illness, unemployment, and old age. The family is viewed as a precious and fragile unit that requires governmental attention and care. In addition to universal health care and significant pension benefits, most European countries provide complete prenatal, delivery, and postpartum expenses, paid maternity/paternity leave (which increases in length with the birth of each child). In addition, in some countries, such as France and Sweden, mothers are paid monthly benefits to defray the cost of the child and can receive "parental education benefits" to allow her to study. They can also obtain subsidized daycare should they attend classes or return to work.

Throughout Europe paid leave of at least twelve weeks is standard (Table 6.3). In Denmark (where 79% of the women work), women are given at least twenty-four weeks of maternity leave, with pay. Subsidized child care is nearly universal. Every country in the European Community guarantees paid maternity leave at between 70% and 100% of a woman's normal salary for between three and five months. France and Belgium provide large cash payments at the birth of a baby to help parents with the added expenses, and eight countries provide monthly family allowances that can continue through college to help with the cost of raising children. In many instances, leave can be shared by either parent, allowing for the parents to choose which one will be the primary caretaker.

In Sweden, a woman who is still nursing upon return to work has the right to take breaks to nurse her infant as she wishes. Often Swedish mothers choose to forgo work in order to stay at home, in which case they can also receive liberal benefits and pay. In addition, Swedish parents have the right to work part-time until a child is eight years old. Norway also has exceptional benefits, allowing eighteen weeks of leave at 100% salary with job protection and two half-hour nursing breaks if the mother is still breast-feeding when she returns to work (if she is a public employee, she can take up to two hours of nursing breaks each day). The father may take fully paid leave for up to two weeks.

The Eastern European countries (Bulgaria, Czechoslovakia, former East Germany, Hungary, Poland, Romania, the former USSR) provide cash maternity benefits under social insurance legislation, with benefits ranging from 65 to 100% of earnings; prohibit dismissal of women during pregnancy and maternity leave; provide extra paid or unpaid leave ranging from a minimum of sixteen weeks in Poland and Romania to twenty-six weeks in Czechoslovakia; and almost all offer nursing breaks to women once they return to the work force. In Bulgaria, working women can extend maternity leave until their children are three years old and still retain their jobs (only a part of this leave is paid).

Almost all Latin American countries provide paid maternity leave at 100% of earnings for twelve weeks or more, and most appear to ensure job security and nursing breaks. Cuba allows eighteen weeks of maternity leave at 100% of earnings with a possible extension to nine months (it is not clear if the extension is on full pay). In three-quarters of the African countries' national maternity policies, there are nursing breaks for working mothers. Mozambique has a particularly progressive policy: maternity leave is only for two months, but two half-hour paid nursing breaks are provided during the working day for a period of six months, and there is paid leave for care of sick children.

Almost all of the Asian/Pacific countries provide paid maternity leave, and over half allow nursing breaks. In China, 100% of earnings are paid by the employer for a total of up to fifty-six days before and after confinement. In India, full pay is provided during maternity leave (social welfare pays the average daily wage, the employer pays the remainder). In a move that is shocking to those who are concerned with overpopulation, rural governments in Japan are offering mothers up to three million yen (about $30,400) for the birth of a *seventh* child. This "Congratulatory Birth Money" is designed to help populate Japan's countryside and to stem the flow of the younger rural population to urban centers.

In many countries, women must take half their leave predelivery and half postdelivery, although they would prefer more time after the birth.

MATERNITY ENTITLEMENTS IN THE UNITED STATES

In a country that continues to view the female labor force participation as voluntary, rather than necessary, it is not surprising that maternity entitlements and child-care provisions are severely lacking in the United States. The majority of working women in America have the worst maternity entitlements: no paid leave, no job security, no lactation breaks, and no explicit provisions for child care.

This has not always been the case. In special circumstances, as in World Wars I and II, women were enticed to join the work force with the offer of crèches, maternity entitlements, lactation breaks, meals on wheels, and child-care centers (one innovative program in Portland, Oregon, even went as far as to make doctors' appointments for children). As soon as the men returned home, however, the women were dismissed, told to go home, and instructed to focus on being good wives and mothers.

In the United States, where individualism reigns and children are viewed as a personal decision, social reformers have focused on equality and parity between genders. Instead of assuming that a man's and a woman's career patterns are inherently different (as European feminists have), the focal point has been proving that women could perform equally in a man's world. Since women working in a man's world are expected to behave like men, maternity and family needs complicate this picture. U.S. women's groups have rejected moves for better maternity protection on the grounds that this will lead to further discrimination. Much female employment, however, is on the fringe economy and workers can be laid off easily. Few unions, not even the predominately female ones, have made maternity entitlement a priority, as they are more concerned to prove themselves in a man's world using men's standards.

Because maternity only affects women and because there has been so much emphasis on being equal with men, no one has known how to classify the process. Battles over employment rights were fought using the Civil Rights Act of 1964, but the courts held that discrimination based on pregnancy was not covered under the umbrella of civil rights. That led Congress to pass the Pregnancy Discrimination Act (PDA) in 1978. The PDA required that employers treat pregnancy and all pregnancy-related concerns the same for all employment-related purposes (including fringe benefit programs) as it did for other disabilities. (The PDA made discrimination illegal, but did nothing to establish any parental entitlements or to foster the combination of working and parenting.)

With pregnancy now classified as a disease, women were entitled to take time off to the extent that they had accrued sick leave. Some employers allowed for leave as a short-term disability. Time off, when it was available, was intended to allow the woman to recover from the physical process of childbirth, not to bond emotionally with the child. (This protected the employer from having to provide leave to fathers or to employees who wanted time off for adopting children.) For female employees fortunate enough to still have a job when they were ready to return from maternity leave, there was very little sympathy—let alone leeway—when family demands interfered with work responsibilities.

In the late 1980s, a "mommy track" was proposed where women could choose to have less work pressure in exchange for fewer options for promotion, but this caused a feminist outcry with concerns such as that all— not just some—jobs should allow for family responsibilities and that the "mommy track" would be imposed on all females as a way of maintaining a "pink collar ghetto." In spite of its view of itself as a world leader and champion of human rights and feminine equality, the United States was the last industrialized nation to establish a national parental leave policy. Until the Family Leave Act was passed in 1993, the United States stood virtually alone among industrialized nations in not mandating family leave. Now that some leave is available, the United States still stands virtually alone among industrialized nations in not mandating paid family leave. Over one hundred countries, including nonindustrialized nations, guarantee workers some form of job-protected, partially paid, maternity-related benefits. It should come as no surprise that the two biggest producers of infant formula, the United States and Switzerland, are the only two industrialized countries without mandated, paid maternity leave.

In response to the growing number of complaints on this matter from constituents, state and local lawmakers began to pass laws mandating various degrees of protection. By the middle of 1992, twenty states as well as the District of Columbia and Dade County, Florida, had passed laws requiring some employers to offer some types of family leave.

At the same time, the National Research Council issued a report, largely financed by the federal government, that argued that parents should be allowed to take as much as a year off from work during the critical early period of their children's lives. The report stressed that parents should not be forced to put their children in second place. Depicting parental leave and quality child care as an investment in the future and a way to build a productive work force, the researchers argued that the costs of not having parental leave are significant, including developmental problems for children, stress on parents trying to combine work and families and lost wages and increased welfare costs for some women if they quit their jobs.

On the national level, Congresswoman Pat Schroeder was leading the battle to put national reforms into place. Back in 1985, she had introduced the Parental and Disability Leave Act. After languishing for years, it finally passed in 1990 only to be vetoed by President Bush. Again in 1992, the bill was approved by Congress only to be again vetoed by President Bush. Finally, in one of his first acts as chief executive, President Clinton signed it into law in the winter of 1993.

The Family and Medical Leave Act, the official U.S. policy on family leave, became law in August 1993, but it is a far cry from setting a new world standard. Over the years the bill was being debated, it was consistently diluted. As introduced in 1985, the act provided for four months of leave and established a commission to study the possibility of paid leave. From its inception, there was well-organized and well-financed opposition from conservatives, business groups, "traditional family" proponents, and the Reagan/Bush White Houses. The opposition had many exaggerated excuses ranging from the practical ("it would be financially crippling") to the philosophical ("government has no place telling businesses how to run their businesses") to the protectional ("it would unfairly result, de facto, in young women being excluded from the job market").

One of the difficulties in getting the Family and Medical Leave Act passed was mustering grassroots support. Pollsters consistently found public backing for a family leave law at over 70%, but supporters were not well organized. As one lobbyist declared, "how many working mothers are in the position of being able to dictate a letter [to Congress] to their secretary?"

The bill that finally emerged requires:

• Employers with fifty or more employees living within a 75-mile radius are required to offer workers up to twelve weeks of unpaid leave after childbirth or adoption; to care for a seriously ill child, spouse, or parent; or a personal illness.

• Employers have to continue health-care coverage during the leave and guarantee employees either the same job or a comparable position upon their return.

• Employers can exempt "key" employees, defined as their highest-paid 10% of the work force and those whose leave would cause economic harm to the employer. Employers may also exempt employees who have worked less than one year or fewer than twenty-five hours a week during the previous year.

While this bill is a positive step and represents good intentions on a serious issue, there are several reasons why it is far from extraordinary. First, only 5% of all companies fit the requirements of those to whom the bill applies. Second, it only covers 50% of all workers. Third, fewer than 40% of working women have sufficient financial protection to enable them to take even a six-week unpaid leave without severe financial consequences. "One of the ironies of this bill," declared Congresswoman Schroeder, "is when I talk to people from other countries, they look at me and say, 'That's all?' And, when I talk to people from this country, they say, 'Oh, my land, that is the most radical thing we have ever heard.'"

Many companies invest money in works of art, sponsorship of sporting and/or cultural events, political donations, and grants and scholarships to academic institutions. They also spend vast sums on prestigious buildings, furnishings, and entertainment as well as on large, well-publicized gifts to charity. Many of these acts are encouraged and then generously rewarded by the government through various tax concessions. Yet businesses insist that they shouldn't have to and could not give a little time off for their employees to take care of their families or to breastfeed their babies, nor could they provide on-site daycare for mothers who wish to breastfeed their babies at work. Equivalent social commitments such as jury or military service cost far more money and decrease a worker's productivity more drastically than breastfeeding a baby, yet there is no opposition to these.

Studies have consistently found that corporate programs that support the family are cost effective. A U.S. General Accounting Office (GAO) study found that family leave policies save employers hiring and training costs, create higher morale, and increase productivity. The GAO has estimated that the legislation would add about 90¢ per worker annually to the cost of benefits—a tiny portion of the roughly $3,500 that companies pay for each employee in medical benefits each year—and that fewer than one in 300 workers would be absent at any one time. A study by the organization 9 to 5 found that the social costs of not providing parental leave are far greater than the costs of regulation and that a policy of parental leave would not interfere with the U.S. ability to compete in the world economy.

Many regional and state laws are more expansive than the national legislation, creating a patchwork of family-leave provisions. The differences in requirements in state and regional rules are confusing for employers and employees alike. Companies with more than twenty-five employees are covered in Maine; the de facto standard in California is four weeks paid disability before, and six weeks paid disability after, delivery *in addition* to unpaid federal family leave; while other states define "family" as including in-laws, and in some places, gay partners. Employers operating in multiple states consider the patchwork of laws mind-boggling, and in many instances employees are unclear on exactly what their rights are.

BREASTFEEDING AT WORK

Religious beliefs, cultural attitudes, and secular laws affect infant feeding patterns, and in many instances, have painted breastfeeding in public as indecent, even obscene, behavior. Negative attitudes to the exposure of the breast have resulted in limiting and, in many instances, cessation of breastfeeding. Instead of hailing the breast for its life-sustaining teleologic purpose, women are made to feel ashamed and embarrassed about the need to expose their breasts in order to nourish their child. This constraint often has excluded breastfeeding women even from educational facilities; only a few programs have allowed mothers to breastfeed and go to school. Unless a woman is able to stay home with the infant at all times or is willing to seek privacy every time the child is hungry, breastfeeding can pose a daunting barrier.

Ironically, the more a woman feels inhibited, restricted, and controlled, the less likely she will be able to breastfeed as breastfeeding requires the woman to be relaxed or the milk refuses to flow. The ease and acceptance of bottle-feeding coupled with extensive advertising by the infant formula industry provides a real temptation to the woman who is not fully convinced of the benefits of breastmilk. Between the demands of the workplace and the cultural taboos of society, breastfeeding is often forced to take a back seat, and what was once the norm has become the exception.

In the United States, there are ample examples of the barriers women face when they try to breastfeed their children. In one incident, a Kansas woman was harassed by a policeman for indecent exposure as she breastfed her infant while sitting quietly in her parked car. Linda Eaton, an Iowa City firefighter, while working on a twenty-four-hour shift, was suspended from her job for breastfeeding her son in 1979. She was sitting in a private room, with her babysitter, during her "personal time" (firefighters are allowed to use this time as they wish—to shower, eat, sleep, read, play cards, etc.). Even though she was nursing when the alarm sounded, she handed her son to the babysitter, prepared herself, and was still aboard the truck before anyone else. The secretary of the firefighter's union was quoted as saying that Linda "is making a mockery of our profession." With the support of the La Leche League International and the National Organization for Women (NOW), Linda went to court and won.

In the fall of 1992, Florida mother Michelle Genz found herself in the center of what was to become a national debate. Inside a shopping mall, Michelle had seated herself in front of a Gap store to nurse her baby. A security guard approached her, demanded to know if she was breastfeeding, and challenged her right to feed her child in public view. Michelle was not only outraged, she was also a freelance writer. She wrote up the incident and placed it in the *Miami Herald Sunday* magazine. Her story was widely read. Miguel DeGrandy, a Cuban-born Republican legislator, decided to do something about it on the political front and introduced legislation to ensure that Michelle's incident would not be repeated. In March 1993, Governor Lawton Chiles signed into law the first state measure in the country guaranteeing women the right to breastfeed in public. Virginia and North Carolina followed suit, passing similar legislation within months. Six states have passed legislation "clarifying" that breastfeeding is not a criminal act (Appendix G).

For the record, there has never actually been a law *against* breastfeeding. Those who harass breastfeeding mothers typically claim that it violates statutes against indecent exposure or obscenity. The Florida legislation specifically states that breastfeeding does not violate prohibitions against "unnatural and lascivious acts or exposure of sexual organs" nor "lewd, lascivious, or indecent conduct in the presence of a child" nor "obscenity" nor "unlawful nudity or sexual conduct . . . irrespective of whether or not the nipple is covered during or incidental to feeding."

The week before Governor Chiles signed the Florida law, a similar incident unfolded in New York. In this case, Liza Habiby was asked to leave a shopping mall in Latham, New York, accused by the mall security guard of exposing herself as she was preparing to nurse her three-month-old son. When other nursing mothers in the area heard of the incident, they organized a nurse-in at the mall—about forty women gathered at the Latham Circle Mall to publicly breastfeed. Within months (May 1994), New York enacted legislation affording legal protection to the act of breastfeeding. Unlike the 1993 laws, which sought to protect a woman's right to breastfeed by exempting the act of breastfeeding from laws governing public nudity and lewd and lascivious behavior, the New York law is tacitly different. It simply states that breastfeeding in public is protected "in any location, public or private, where the mother is otherwise authorized to be, irrespective of whether or not the nipple of the mother's breast is covered during or incidental to the breastfeeding." Activists in other states are now examining how to get their legislatures to introduce similar bills as a means of bringing breastfeeding to public discussion.

Clearly, the positive outcome to these small incidents is due in part to increased public awareness of the benefits of breastfeeding, but both stories are also tributes to the Michelles and Lizas of the world who each decided to take action against what they perceived was an injustice. Had Michelle and Liza simply gone home and vowed never to breastfeed in public again, countless women would still lack protection and millions of people would have escaped discussion of the issue (both laws were covered extensively on talk shows).

There are still no national laws to protect breastfeeding mothers, let alone breastfeeding employees. However, these events may be the first indicators that the pendulum is now swinging the other way. The same month that the New York legislation became law, President Clinton voted to impose restrictions on infant formula promotion (see "The United States Embraces the Code" in chapter 5). Making clear his commitment to encouraging breastfeeding in the United States, he joined an unprecedented worldwide consensus to support the WHO/UNICEF International Code of Marketing of Breastmilk Substitutes. These actions demonstrate a new American commitment to the promotion and protection of breastfeeding.

Planning to return to work when the baby is less than one year old is a major consideration in choosing whether to breastfeed or bottle-feed. Early return to work is often a deterrent to breastfeeding, but it does not have to be. For example, in Norway, women who go back to work within the

Figure 6.2
Combining Work and Family Life

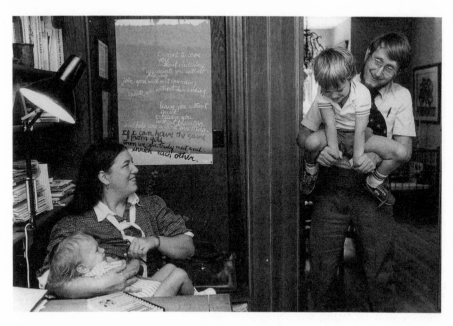

This father brings the baby to the mother's office for a nursing break. *Photo courtesy*: Sally Strosahl, Courtesy: La Leche League International.

first twelve months after a birth breastfeed *more* than those who stay at home. In contrast, in the United States, maternal employment is often cited as a major contributing factor for the decline in the duration of breastfeeding. Increased distance from work as well as early return to work have been associated with a higher frequency of formula or mixed feeding.

In the United States, weaning before six months of age is highest when the mother returns to full-time employment before the infant is sixteen weeks old. Furthermore, when the mother returns to work after birth, this appears to have a greater effect on weaning than the number of hours per week she works (although part-time workers are more likely than full-time workers to nurse their infants longer than one year). In one study, non-white women were five times more likely than whites to wean their babies before twenty-six weeks. Of the women who did continue breastfeeding after returning to work, none reported breastfeeding influenced their work negatively.

The combination of returning to work and feeding a child does not have to pose a problem (Figure 6.2). On-site day care and lactation breaks can be combined to allow women to take care of their job and nourish their children. Sweden, Norway, Brazil, and Honduras permit workers with new-

Figure 6.3
Permission to Breastfeed

Honduras Breastfeeding Authorization Letter

The undersigned physician, in charge of the Well Baby Clinic affirms that Mrs.

_____ ,

number _____ had a baby on _____ and is breastfeeding.
Therefore, I request that your company extend to her a paid hour for
breastfeeding which is supported by Article No. 140 in the Labor Code.

Translation of a permission form developed to enable breastfeeding factory employees to take lactation breaks. *Courtesy*: Judy Canahuatis.

borns to return to work and continue breastfeeding through the provision of on-site nurseries and lactation breaks. In Honduras, medical certificates are given to factory workers to enable them to utilize lactation breaks (Figure 6.3). Employers felt certification would prevent abuse of the privilege by non-lactating women.

Measures conducive to the promotion of breastfeeding have been advocated by a number of organizations, including the International Pediatric Association (IPA) and the International Confederation of Midwives (ICM). IPA recommends that the workplace provide facilities for breastfeeding, modify the work day of breastfeeding women, extend maternity leave to permit breastfeeding, and provide appropriate allowances for nursing mothers. ICM at its 1984 International Congress issued statements that it recognizes "the right of all babies to be breastfed for at least the first six months of life" and stressed the importance of breastfeeding in developing countries in reducing malnutrition, morbidity, and mortality.

Although the U.S. Surgeon General has strongly endorsed the concept of breastfeeding and hopes to increase breastfeeding rates, very little has been done to promote it, and many women feel that breastfeeding and employment are currently incompatible. Realistically, a working woman has two choices if she wants to nurse and work: she can have the baby cared for near her job so she can feed during break times (which is difficult, as many daycare facilities do not accept infants nor are they necessarily close to places of employment) or she can express breastmilk several times a day (either manually or with a breast pump), refrigerate it, and bring it home to the babysitter to feed to the baby during working hours. Both scenarios require the employee to have some flexibility in her daily schedule and a

Table 6.4
Obstacles to Breastfeeding for Working Mothers

- Early return to work

- Limited opportunities for part-time work

- Distance to work

- Type of work

- Job security

- Stringent work schedule

- Hostile attitudes from management and peers

- Hostile attitude of health care workers

- Lack of suitable day care

- Low status of women in the workforce

place where she can have privacy and access to refrigeration. An increasing number of women would like to breastfeed but cannot because no time or place is available for this during working hours. Even if the mother is committed to continuing the breastfeeding relationship, many employers don't see breastfeeding as a function of the workplace. Table 6.4 lists the common obstacles to breastfeeding in the workplace.

However, some women have taken steps to challenge the system and alter this. Such was the experience last year of Teresa Riegal, an $8 per hour production line worker at Chrysler, who mistakenly assumed she would be able to pump milk for her baby when she returned to work. She asked her boss to allow her to lengthen her fifteen-minute breaks so she would have sufficient time to pump breastmilk during the workday. Chrysler refused and only offered to extend her unpaid leave. She sued for discrimination, contending that the company was forcing her to choose between her baby and her job. Chrysler defended itself saying that it had to treat workers equally under its union contract and that it could not shut down an entire assembly line for one employee. As the trial date approached, the company hired a lactation consultant to help her cut the time she needed to pump and to set up a room for that purpose. Teresa was out of work for nine months because of the dispute before the suit was settled out of court.

While the pumping battle was being fought in Michigan, another battle was brewing in Florida. Judy Deelay, a traffic court clerk, claimed she had to sit in her car, in 100°F heat, after she was officially reprimanded by her supervisor for combining her breaks to pump breastmilk in a rarely used workroom. The latest report is that a grievance committee rescinded her supervisor's reprimand and the county employees have agreed to develop a countywide policy on breastfeeding.

In the United States, it is often the exceptional, highly educated, and decidedly determined mother who manages to combine employment with breastfeeding. It does not have to be this way. The Los Angeles Department of Water and Power has had a program running for over five years (developed with Medela, Inc., a leading manufacturer of breast pumps) that has become a nationwide model. Estimates indicate that the department has saved nearly $5 for every $1 spent on the breastfeeding program, citing dramatic reductions in worker absenteeism and the company's health care costs, about one-third of which are infant related. A two-year study of employee's breastfed babies found that only 59% had been ill at least once, compared with 93% of the formula-fed infants.

Some corporations have established lactation rooms to make it easier for breastfeeding workers. Chicago-based Amoco Corporation decided to supply lightweight, miniaturized breast pumps to nursing mothers who must travel, to eliminate the need for them to carry around bulkier, heavier machines. Many federal offices have established pumping rooms and daycare facilities. The need for women to combine pumping and work has not escaped the Clinton White House. For the first time in White House history, a member of the executive staff, the Presidential Assistant for Political Affairs, was given a breast pump so that she could continue to provide her child with breastmilk and manage her career.

A recent study conducted by Rona Cohen, at the University of California, Los Angeles, found that when an employer provided space, equipment, and a lactation consultant, 75% of the survey participants were able to breastfeed their infants for six months or more. In some cases, the firms provide only the space with employees donating and raising money to buy pumps and a refrigerator (large hospital-grade pumps are much more effective than small, portable pumps, so women who are pumping regularly much prefer access to these larger, more expensive units).

One community hospital in New Jersey provides time off and facilities for nursing mothers to pump their breasts during the work day. The hospital also allows mothers to transfer to a location closer to home in order to go home and nurse their infants during breaks if they wished. These mothers nurse for longer and are more likely to continue nursing after return to employment. In a study of working women in four Boston city hospitals, it was found that continued breastfeeding was attributed to a flexible work schedule and a sympathetic boss. IBM instituted a new policy of offering employees up to three years of unpaid leave for a "serious reason," including care of a new child. While employees do not get paid, they do continue receiving company-paid benefits and are assured of a job when they return. Southern New England Telephone is now offering up to one year of unpaid leave to care for a newborn or newly adopted child with a guarantee of a job upon the employee's return. The company says that the leave program is cost effective and has a positive effect on productivity.

When corporate policy does not support breastfeeding, creative solutions might make the difference. In some cases, breastmilk banks have been established so that nurseries can get milk for working mothers' infants (although it is not necessarily the mother's milk). Some companies have purchased electric breast pumps for their employees to use at work. In addition, job sharing can give women increased flexibility and the ability to work part-time, just as cross-nursing can allow full-time workers to have their children receive breastmilk exclusively (a case in point is that of a social worker and a teacher, both with infants; the teacher worked during the day and the social worker in the evening, and each woman breastfed both babies when they were home). Isolated creative solutions, however, should not be the only solutions.

There are interesting lessons to be learned from an accident in Mozambique. A cashew nut processing plant established an on-site daycare center, well housed and well staffed, for the children of their employees. Burglars stole the bottles used to feed the babies. Rather than ordering more, management allowed the mothers to breastfeed their babies for two periods of a half-hour per shift and moved mothers to the part of the factory closest to the crèche. Breastfeeding was encouraged and mothers were allowed to work in pairs for mutual support. The center is a tremendous success and the women are considered contented and productive workers. This is in striking contrast to another daycare center at a Mozambican cotton factory, where babies are bottle-fed with breastmilk substitutes. At that facility, similarly well housed and well staffed, there are constant problems with diarrhea and malnutrition.

The trend to meet the needs of new mothers has been bolstered by a number of studies that have proven that family and medical leave policies are good business. The more scarce certain types of workers are and the higher the costs of training new ones, the more financially important it becomes to meet the needs of current employees. Daycare has become a very attractive fringe benefit. A Boston University report to the Ford Foundation, summarizing more than a decade of research, found that family-friendly policies, particularly on-site child care, increases workers' job satisfaction and morale and reduces absenteeism, turnover, and tardiness. A 1982 tax break for employers providing daycare facilities for employees has helped provide an incentive. Many companies are concluding that unless they help their working parents—who represent the next generation of management—to meet family responsibilities, they run the risk of losing them to competitors who do.

Some corporations have started offering on-site daycare facilities, the most progressive of which offer flextime and provide private rooms for nursing so mothers can breastfeed on demand. Law firms are increasingly allowing women attorneys employed full-time to return to work part-time after a birth. Another increasing trend is to let employees make their own child-care arrangements, but to offer backup care. Time Warner, Inc., opened a free, emergency daycare center in the lobby of its corporate head-quarters in New York City in November 1992. The center serves as many as thirty children a day from ages six months to twelve years. When a babysitter is sick or on vacation, when a school is closed, or extra time has to be worked, employees can take their kids to the backup center. Arnold & Porter, a Washington, DC, law firm, opened a backup center on its premises in 1989 that is open 363 days a year. The firm estimated the center saved $500,000 in attorney time in 1992 that would have been lost because staff would have been forced to stay home. There are also a number of sick children's centers opening in Westchester, New York, to care for mildly ill children (cold, flu, etc.). Sick care and backup centers save money in lost productivity from absenteeism, relieve parental stress, and promote em-ployee loyalty.

The needs of the family are increasingly being weighed in employer pol-icies. In a big move, the federal government has proposed to allow em-ployees to use up to five days of sick leave each year to care for a child, spouse, or parent; currently, employees can only use sickleave for their own illnesses. While employers examine their policies, so do potential employ-ees. *Working Mother* magazine publishes a well-watched list each year of the nation's best companies for employed mothers. The 1993 list named eighty-five firms, a mixture of small and large companies, more than half of which have their own child-care centers. Not to leave out half the family, *Child* magazine publishes its own "Best Companies for Dads" listing each year.

The progress in developing work-friendly workplaces is impressive, yet programs designed to meet the needs of working parents are still very much the exception. It is hoped that as news of the success of such programs travels, more options will proliferate. Recent adaptations of U.S. businesses to a changing work force do not mean that the needs of all, or even most, women are adequately met. Many parents are still forced to choose between their families and their jobs. Where maternity entitlements exist, they may be modified or dispensed with at the discretion of the employer. It is un-reasonable not to promote breastfeeding when it is so clearly the superior infant feeding method, but it is unreasonable to promote breastfeeding in a society without also providing working women an adequate opportunity to do so. In South Africa, for example, trade unions have served as the vehicle for women to demand entitlements. International organizations, such as the World Alliance for Breastfeeding Action (WABA), are promot-ing measures to improve the environment in the workplace for breastfeed-ing. If we are going to increase the current percentages of nursing mothers in the work force, significant steps need to be taken to make the work

Table 6.5
Promoting Breastfeeding in the Workplace

CONSTRAINTS	SOLUTIONS
Attitudes: cultural, employer, employee	Education Child-care centers, information, and referral services Support

Insufficient national protections	National health maternity policy with
	   guarantee of job reinstatement, nursing
	   breaks, and paid leave

Time—schedules	Nursing breaks Flextime Part-time Job-sharing Option to work from home
Place—facilities	On-site daycare Employer tax incentive for providing facilities, breast pumps, refrigerators Safe, clean environment
Expense	National Insurance Fund and/or employer contribution Daycare subsidies
Lack of organization	Committed trade unions Committed elected officials Committed policy planners

environment more safe and supportive. Table 6.5 lists some of the constraints and solutions in promoting breastfeeding in the workplace.

Just as the two women who were harassed for breastfeeding in shopping malls stood their ground, it is the actions and attitudes of individual women that are driving changes in employer-provided lactation facilities. Women who consider breastfeeding a necessity and a right, not a luxury, have propelled much of the energy. They compare their right to pump to the diabetic worker who doesn't have to ask permission to check blood sugar levels and/or administer insulin. Assuming breastfeeding is a medical necessity and that it does not need to conflict with work schedules or requirements is the first step. Other women have found it very helpful to compare their time away from their desks for pumping to cigarette smokers who take time away for smoking breaks. This comparison is increasingly relevant since more and more work environments are smoke-free, necessitating smokers to be physically absent from the work environment in order to cater to their nicotine dependency. Pointing out that a woman who goes off to pump spends no more time away from her desk than smokers spend smoking can help diffuse tension about the absences.

Modern-day realities translate into stress, insecurity, and child neglect, setting the stage for an encyclopedia of problems, both present and future. The question is not "What do women want?" or even "What do working women want?" The question is "What do families need?" We know the answer. Families need flexible work schedules; affordable, safe, nearby child care; illness-related or emergency child care; parental leave options; affordable health care and quality schools; financial assistance for children and medical expenses; and sympathetic supervisors. In this time of single parent and two worker families, the conflict between parenting and work is a significant problem; better federal, state, and local laws to protect the family must be a priority.

Appendix A

Organizations Working to Promote Breastfeeding

ACTION FOR CORPORATE ACCOUNTABILITY

Action for Corporate Accountability, a nonprofit organization, alerts the public to corporate practices which cause infant death and disease and takes direct action to stop these practices. Action coordinates the boycott against Nestlé and American Home Products in the United States and is a member of the International Baby Food Action Network (IBFAN).

910 17th Street, NW
#413
Washington, DC 20006
Telephone: 202-776-0595; Fax: 202-776-0599

BABY MILK ACTION (BMA)

This is a nonprofit organization that aims to halt the commercial promotion of bottle-feeding and to protect and promote good infant nutrition. BMA is a member of IBFAN and produces four newsletters a year.

23 St. Andrew's Street
Cambridge, England CB2 3AX
Telephone: (44-223) 464-420; Fax: (44-223) 464-417

CHILD HEALTH FOUNDATION

This is a U.S.-based, nonprofit group concerned with improving child health. They produce programs for diarrheal disease control and prevention and promote breastfeeding in this context. They produce a newsletter four times a year.

10630 Little Patuxent Parkway
Suite 325, Century Plaza

P.O. Box 1205, Columbia, MD 21044
Telephone: 301-596-4514; Fax: 410-992-5641

CLEARINGHOUSE ON INFANT FEEDING AND MATERNAL NUTRITION

This project is funded by USAID's Office on Nutrition at the American Public Health Association. It provides information and support to practitioners in developing countries. It maintains a breastfeeding database and produces a newsletter (available in English, French, and Spanish) three times a year.

Clearinghouse, c/o APHA
1015 15th Street, NW
Washington, DC 20005
Telephone: 202-789-5611; Fax: 202-789-5661

GENEVA INFANT FEEDING ASSOCIATION (GIFA)

This group, a member of IBFAN, produces *Breastfeeding Briefs*, a collection of new research findings on breastfeeding. It is available in English, French, Spanish, and Portuguese.

Box 157
1211 Geneva 19
Switzerland
Telephone: (41-22) 798-9164; Fax: (41-22) 798-4441

HEALTHY MOTHERS, HEALTHY BABIES

This is a coalition of over ninety national professional, voluntary, and nongovernmental organizations for public education to improve maternal and child health. There are a number of committees, including one on breastfeeding. Each committee produces education materials and programs.

409 12th Street, SW
Washington, DC 20024-2188
Telephone: 202-863-2458; Fax: 202-484-5107

HEALTHY MOTHERS/HEALTHY BABIES COALITION

This is the group responsible for the U.S. Baby-Friendly Hospital Initiative Feasibility Study.

700 W. 40th Street, Suite 325
Baltimore, MD 21211
Telephone: 410-243-9426; Fax: 410-243-3163

INFANT FEEDING ACTION COALITION (INFACT) CANADA

INFACT is a nongovernmental, nonprofit organization that supports and protects breastfeeding in Canada. They have a breastfeeding information clearinghouse, produce a newsletter, and monitor government policies and industry compliance with WHO/UNICEF directives. They also produce educational programs for the public and health care professionals.

10 Trinity Square
Toronto, Canada M5G 1B1
Telephone: 416-595-9819; Fax: 416-598-1432

INSTITUTE FOR REPRODUCTIVE HEALTH—BREASTFEEDING DIVISION

This is the first WHO collaborative center for breastfeeding. The Institute conducts research and provides information on birth spacing and breastfeeding. They provide technical support and produce educational materials, including videos and slides.

Georgetown University Medical Center
2115 Wisconsin Avenue, NW
Washington, DC 20007
Telephone: 202-687-6846; Fax: 202-687-1392

INTERNATIONAL BABY FOOD ACTION NETWORK (IBFAN)

This is a coalition of more than 140 citizen groups in 70 developing and industrialized nations. IBFAN works for better child health and nutrition through the promotion of breastfeeding and the elimination of irresponsible marketing of infant foods, feeding bottles, and teats. There are IBFAN groups all over the world. Some central offices are:

IBFAN/International Organization of Consumers' Unions
P.O. Box 1045
10830 Penang, Malaysia
Telephone: (60-4) 371-1396; Fax: (60-4) 366-506

IBFAN International Baby Food Action Network—Africa
Mbabane, Swaziland
Telephone: 268-45006; Fax: 268-44246

INTERNATIONAL LACTATION CONSULTANT ASSOCIATION (ILCA)

ILCA is a nonprofit organization which provides education, communication, networking and mutual support for lactation consultants and other health workers caring for breastfeeding women, infants and children. ILCA sponsors a quarterly journal, a bimonthly newsletter and other lactation related publications.

200, N. Michigan Avenue, Suite 300,
Chicago IL 60601-3821.
Telephone: 312-541-1271; Fax: 312-541-1271

LA LECHE LEAGUE INTERNATIONAL

LLLI is a nonprofit service organization that offers information and support in sixty countries around the world for mothers who choose to breastfeed their babies. The organization also provides educational opportunities for health care professionals and lay counselors. LLLI is recognized as the world's foremost authority on breastfeeding and produces (in a variety of languages) books, articles, pamphlets, and three newsletters—one for parents, one for accredited leaders, and one for health care professionals.

1400 N. Meacham Road
P.O. Box 4079
Schaumburg, IL 60173
Telephone: 708-519-7730; Fax: 708-519-0035

NATIONAL CAPITAL LACTATION CENTER

This Center is comprised of an interdisciplinary team of professionals who provide a complete range of breastfeeding services. They offer educational programs and run the Community Human Milk Bank, which provides pasteurized donor breastmilk, by doctor's prescription, wherever it is needed.

Georgetown University Medical Center
3800 Reservoir Road, NW
Washington, DC 20007
Telephone: 202-784-MILK (6455); Fax: 202-784-2575

UNITED NATIONS INTERNATIONAL CHILDREN'S EDUCATION FUND (UNICEF)

UNICEF is a United Nations specialized agency concerned with a range of activities in the developing world focused on child health. Provides training and programs in the developing world, and produces a variety of publications and audiovisual materials.

3 United Nations Plaza
The United Nations
New York, NY 10017

WELLSTART INTERNATIONAL

Wellstart is an independent nonprofit organization. The mission of the organization is the global promotion of healthy families through the global promotion of breastfeeding. The centerpiece of Wellstart's mission is the education of health care providers and policymaker leadership followed by working closely with these colleagues to help them develop and undertake national breastfeeding promotion programs appropriate to their own situations. The organization has a number of projects including Wellstart Expanded Breastfeeding Promotion (EPB) which was established for breastfeeding research evaluation and now is in its final phase.

4062 First Avenue
San Diego, CA 92103
Telephone: 619-298-7979; Fax: 619-294-7787

WOMEN'S INTERNATIONAL PUBLIC HEALTH NETWORK (WIPHN)

This is a grassroots nonprofit organization of women in public health and health-related areas working to improve the health, nutrition, and status of women globally. WIPHN produces quarterly newsletters.

7100 Oak Forest Lane
Bethesda, MD 20817
Telephone: 301-469-9210; Fax: 301-469-8423

WORLD ALLIANCE FOR BREASTFEEDING ACTION (WABA)

WABA is a global network of organizations and individuals who believe breastfeeding is a right of all children and mothers; their mission is to protect, promote, and support this right. Through World Breastfeeding Week (the first week of August, each year), WABA has focused annually on special initiatives including The Baby-Friendly Hospital Initiative, The Mother Friendly Workplace Initiative, and Making the Code Work. The organization monitors violations of the WHO/UNICEF International Code of Marketing Breastmilk Substitutes.

P.O. Box 1200
10850 Penang, Malaysia
Telephone: (60-4) 884-816; Fax: (60-4) 872-2655

WORLD HEALTH ORGANIZATION (WHO)

This is a specialized agency of the United Nations providing services to governments and technical services throughout the world. WHO produces a variety of materials, including some on breastfeeding.

20 Avenue Appia
CH-1211 Geneva 27
Switzerland

Appendix B

Recommended Reading
and Resource List

BOOKS

The Politics of Breastfeeding, Gabrielle Palmer, Pandora Press, 1994, $16.95.
   A provocative book challenging the assumptions of a bottle-feeding culture.
The Nature of Birth and Breastfeeding, Michel Odent, Bergin and Garvey, 1992,
   $16.95.
A fascinating book challenging western assumptions on childbirth and breast-
feeding.
Breastfeeding Matters, What We Need to Know, Maureen Minchin, Alma
   Publications and Allen and Unwin, Alfredton, Australia, 1989, $19.95.
   An interesting book covering the political and the personal side of breastfeeding.
Beyond the Breast-Bottle Controversy, Penny Van Esterik, Rutgers University Press,
   1989, $13.00.
A book that explores how formula-feeding is embedded in the problems of urban
poverty and the medicalization of infant feeding.
Breaking the Rules, Andrew Radford and Maaike Arts, International Baby Food
   Action Network/International Organization of Consumer's Unions, 1994,
   $6.00. Available from Action, 129 Church St., New Haven, CT 06510.
   A worldwide report on violations of the WHO/UNICEF International Code of
Marketing of Breastmilk Substitutes, indexed both by country and company.
The Mother Zone, Marni Jackson, Henry Holt & Co., 1994, $12.95.
   A warm and witty book in which the author describes the experience of being a
mother.
Breastfeeding Pure & Simple, Gwen Gotsch, La Leche League International, Frank-
   lin Park, IL, 1994, $8.95.
   A good book with basic information, guides you through the early months of
nursing.
The Womanly Art of Breastfeeding, La Leche League International, Plume, 1991,
   $10.95.

The classic book on breastfeeding (an abridged version of this book is available in a 2-cassette audio set for $9.95).

Bestfeeding: Getting Breastfeeding Right for You, Mary Renfrew, Chloe Fisher, and Suzanne Arms, Celestial Arts, 1990, $12.95.

A good, basic how-to book for new mothers.

The Complete Book of Breastfeeding, Marvin S. Eiger, M.D., and Sally Wendkos Olds, Workman Publishing, 1987, $8.95.

A thorough how-to book.

The Breastfeeding Answer Book, Nancy Mohrbacher and Julie Stock, La Leche League International, 1991, $32.95.

This book was designed for lactation professionals, it explores a broad spectrum of information and deals with all types of breastfeeding questions.

Breastfeeding: A Guide for the Medical Profession, Ruth A. Lawrence, C.V. Mosby Company, 1994, $60.00.

The standard-bearer of breastfeeding books for the medical profession.

AUDIO AND VIDEO TAPES

Protecting Infant Health: Making the Code Work, INFACT, 1994, 30 minutes, $20.00. Available from INFACT, 10 Trinity Square, Toronto, Canada, M5G 1B1, 416-595-9819, 416-591-9355—fax.

A brand new guide to the Code, suitable for provoking discussion and providing background for action groups/health workers.

Formula for Disaster, Action for Corporate Accountability, 1992, 18 minutes, $5.00/rental, $25.00/purchase. Available from Action, 129 Church St., New Haven, CT 06510, 203-787-0061, 203-787-3908—fax.

An exposé of the role infant formula companies have played in destroying breast-feeding cultures within developing countries and how that has led to a yearly death toll of over one million infants.

A Healthier Baby by Breastfeeding, La Leche League International, 1992, 20 minutes, $19.95. Available from LLLI, 1400 N. Meacham Road, P.O. Box 4079, Schaumburg, IL 60173, 708-519-7730, 708-519-0035—fax.

A video to help you get started breastfeeding.

The Formula Fix, Australian Broadcasting Commission, 1989, 45 minutes, $25.00. Available from INFACT, 10 Trinity Square, Toronto, Canada, M5G 1B1, 416-595-9819, 416-591-9355—fax.

A video that examines the problems of formula-feeding.

The Womanly Art of Breastfeeding, La Leche League International, 1988, two audio cassettes, $9.95. Available from LLLI, 1400 N. Meacham Road, P.O. Box 4079, Schaumburg, IL 60173, 708-519-7730, 708-519-0035—fax.

The classic book on breastfeeding in an abridged audio version.

When Breasts Are Bad for Business, Baby Milk Action, 1985, 30 minutes, $25.00. Available from INFACT, 10 Trinity Square, Toronto, Canada, M5G 1B1, 416-595-9819, 416-591-9355—fax.

A video that examines the financial incentives for formula manufacturers to encourage women to abandon breastfeeding—and how to counter them.

BREASTFEEDING MERCHANDISE, POSTERS, AND SO ON

Baby Milk Action sells breastfeeding and Nestlé boycott postcards, greeting cards, T-shirts, mugs, and bumper stickers, as well as books and video tapes.

23 St. Andrew's Street
Cambridge, England CB2 3AX
0223-464420, 0223-464417—fax

Action for Corporate Accountability sells T-shirts, posters, bumper stickers, and buttons, as well as books and video tapes.

c/o Community Nutrition Institute
202-776-0595, 202-776-0599—fax

La Leche League International has an extensive mail-order catalog with books, video tapes, cassette tapes, posters, jewelry, tote bags, infant carriers, breast pumps, and more.

1400 N. Meacham Road
P.O. Box 4079
Schaumburg, IL 60173
708-519-7730, 708-519-0035—fax

INFACT sells T-shirts and posters, as well as books and video tapes.

10 Trinity Square
Toronto, Canada M5G 1B1
416-595-9819, 416-591-9355—fax

National Capital Lactation Center runs programs and workshops for health professionals and sells videos, brochures, posters, and articles.

Georgetown University Medical Center
3800 Reservoir Road, NW
Washington, DC 20007
202-784-MILK (6455), 202-784-2575—fax

Women's International Public Health Network sells books, T-shirts, calendars, and the *Test Your Breastfeeding IQ Quiz* (excerpted from this book).

7100 Oak Forest Lane
Bethesda, MD 20817
301-469-9210, 301-469-8423—fax

Appendix C

U.S. Infant Formula Recalls, 1982–1994

Class I: A product whose use may cause serious health consequences
Class II: A product which may cause medically reversible health conditions
Class III: A product whose use is not likely to cause medically adverse health effects

Problem	Product recalled	Class	Date
Klebsiella and pseudomona contaminants	Nursoy concentrate (Wyeth Labs)	II	1994
Salmonella contamination	Soyalac (Nutricia Inc.)	I	1993
Glass contamination	Nutramigen (Mead Johnson)	II	1993
Peeling can lining	Isomil Soy Formula with iron concentrate (Ross Laboratories)	III	1993
Bacterial contamination	I-Soylac Concentrated infant formula (Loma Linda Foods)	I	1990
Deficient in Vitamin D, below label claim for Vitamin K	Similac PM60/40 low iron infant formula (Ross Labs)	III	1989
Unfit appearance, didn't pass through bottle nipple	Carnation Good Nature infant formula for infants over 6 months (Nestlé)	III	1989

Problem	Product recalled	Class	Date
Deficient in Vitamin D	Nutramigen iron fortified protein hydrolysate formula (Mead Johnson)	III	1989
Progressive Vitamin A degradation	Soyalac powder (Loma Linda Foods)	III	1986
Curdling, discoloration	SMA Ready to Feed (Wyeth Labs)	II	1986
Superpotent Vitamin A levels	Gerber Meat Base formula with iron (Gerber)	II	1985
Deficient in folacin, Vitamin D, and zinc; marked in violation of Infant Formula Act	Kama-Mil powder (Kama Nutritional Products)	I	1985
Deficient in folacin, Vitamin D, and zinc; marked in violation of Infant Formula Act	Nutra-milk powder formula (Mead Johnson)	I	1985
Pamphlet erroneously suggests Edensoy may be used as substitute for human milk or infant formula	"Edensoy" pamphlet (Eden Foods)	I	1985
Deficient in copper and linoleic acid; not in compliance with Food, Drug and Cosmetic Act	Cow & Gate Improved Modified Infant Formula (Cow and Gate)	II	1985

Problem	Product recalled	Class	Date
Deficient in copper and linoleic acid; not in compliance with Food, Drug and Cosmetic Act	Lactogen with iron (Nestlé)	III	1985
Glass particles (from bottle chipping)	5% glucose water (Ross Labs)	II	1985
Overprocessed, lumpy, brown; unfit for human consumption	Similac with iron (Ross Labs)	II	1985
Deficient in Vitamin A	Soyalac Powder Milk Free Fortified Soy Formula (Loma Linda Foods)	II	1983
Copper below Infant Formula Act requirement; thiamine and Vitamin B^6 less than stated on the label	Naturlac Infant formula (Filmore Foods)	II	1983
Deficient in B^6	Nursoy Concentrated Liquid (Wyeth Laboratories)	I	1982
Deficient in B^6; less than stated on the label	All ready-to-feed: SMA iron fortified, SMA powder, SMA E-Z Nurser (Wyeth Labs)	I	1982

Source: All data derived from the *FDA Enforcement Report*, June 1994, Press Office, Food and Drug Administration, HFI-20, 5600 Fishers Lane, Rockville, MD 20857; and from M.J. Walker, "A Fresh Look at the Risks of Artificial Infant Feeding," *Journal of Human Lactation*, 9(2) (1993).

Appendix D

Boycott Information

In 1977, a consumer boycott was initiated against Nestlé in response to their formula marketing practices in third-world nations. The aim of the boycott was to force Nestlé to end practices detrimental to breastfeeding, specifically for Nestlé to halt all promotion of baby milk, including milk nurses, free samples, and advertising. The boycott gained momentum in the United States and quickly spread to Canada, Europe, and New Zealand.

After the passage of the WHO/UNICEF International Code of Marketing of Breastmilk Substitutes in 1981, Nestlé stated that they would direct their employees to abide by this Code. Later, Nestlé signed an agreement with the International Nestlé Boycott Committee in which they agreed to develop marketing policies that were consistent with the intent of the Code and to follow guidelines to be established by UNICEF and WHO on the distribution of free supplies. As a result, the boycott was suspended in early 1984, and, after a six-month test period, it was officially halted.

However, in response to continuing widespread and egregious violations of the International Code, Action for Corporate Accountability reinstated the boycott against Nestlé in October 1988. The International Nestlé Boycott Committee now has coordinating groups in 14 countries. The boycott was also expanded to target American Home Products (the second largest manufacturer of infant formula in the world) by groups in the United States, Philippines, Australia, and Canada.

Organizers vow that the boycott will continue this time until sustained monitoring shows that these two companies have ended all promotion of bottle-feeding, especially those that promote the purchase or use of infant formula, follow-up milks, feeding bottles, teats, and any other product that replaces breastmilk. After the last boycott experience, organizers have decided to maintain the boycott until compliance is verified by monitoring for an eighteen-month period.

The boycott is being coordinated in this country by Action (Action for Corporate Accountability in Connecticut (see Appendix A for the complete address). Action has supplied a complete list of the boycotted products (as of 4/95), which is reproduced below.

A more detailed history of the boycott and the WHO Code can be found in chapter 5, "The Global Search for Formula Sales."

NESTLÉ PRODUCTS

Candies and Ice Creams

After Eights

Baby Ruth

Bit O' Honey

Breyer's Ice Cream

Butterfinger

Chunky

DeMet's turtles

Goobers

Harry Lunden candies (used in fundraising)

Heath ice cream bars

Katherine Beich candies (used in fundraising)

Kit Kat

Nestlé Alpine White chocolate

Nestlé BonBons Ice Cream Nuggets

Nestlé Cool Creations Frozen Treats

Nestlé Crunch

Oh Henry!

Pearsons Nips

Perugina Chocolates

Rountree candies

Smarties

Snocaps

Sunmark Raisinets

Other Nestlé-owned Products

Buitoni (pasta and canned goods)

Chase & Sanborn coffee

Contadina canned tomato products

Hills Brother's Coffees

Libby's canned vegetables

Libby's fruit nectars

Libby's Juicy Juice

MJB (rice and rice mixes)

Maggi soups & seasonings

Nescafé

Nestea Instant Tea

Nestlé Cocoa

Nestlé Quik

Nestlé Toll House Chocolate Chips

Taster's Choice Coffees

Carnation Products

Carnation evaporated milk

Carnation hot cocoa mix

Carnation institutional products

Carnation powdered skimmed milk

Coffee-mate non-dairy creamer

Dr. Ballard's dog foods

Stouffer Food Products

Stouffer frozen entrees, including

   Lean Cuisine

   Stouffer's Dinner Supreme

Stouffer Restaurants

Borels

Cheese Cellar

Chicago

J.B. Winberie

James Tavern

One Nation

Parker's Lighthouse

Pier East

The Roxy

Rusty Scupper

The Whole Grain

Bottled Waters

Arrowhead

Calistoga

Dear Park

Great Bear

Ice Mountain

Oasis

Ozarka

Perrier

Poland Springs

Utopia

Vittel

Zephyr Hills

Wines and Other Beverages

Beringer

Chateau Souverain

Napa Ridge

Wine World

Cosmetics

Alcon Laboratories

L'Oreal

Warner

Pet Foods

Alpo (canned and dry) cat and dog
   foods

Chef's Blend dry cat food

Fancy Feast canned cat food

Friskies (canned and dry) cat and dog
   foods

Mighty Dog canned dog food

Drugs/Medications

Advil

Anacin and Anacin 3

Anbesol topical anesthetic

Arthritis Pain Formula

Centrum vitamins

Chapstick

Compound W

Dermoplast

Dimatab

Dristan

Fibercom laxatives

Medicated Cleaning Pads

Momentum

Norplant

Preparation H

Primatene

Riopan and Bisodol antacids

Robitussin

Sleepeze

Household and Cleaning Products

Aerowax

Antrol insecticides

Black Flag

Easy-Off Glass Cleaner

Easy-On Speed Starch

Gulf Lite

Kwik Lite

Old English Furniture Care Products

Sani-Flush

3-in-One-Oils

Wizard Aerosol/Decoratives/Dry
   Breezes

Wizard Charcoal Lighter

Woolite

Zud

Personal Care Products

Clearblue pregnancy test kit

Clearplan ovulation test kit

Denorex

Freezone

Neet

Outgro

Q-tip glass thermometers

Semicid

Today condoms and sponges

Foods, Seasonings, and Condiments

Chef Boyardee food products

Dennison's Chili

Franklin Crunch 'n Munch

G. Washington products

Gulden's Mustard

Jiffy Popcorn

Luck's country and ranch style beans

Mamma Leone's Pasta supreme

Pam cooking sprays

Polaner jams & jellies

AHP Brands

A.H. Robbins

American Home Foods

American Home Products

Sherwood Medical

Whitehall Labs

Wyeth-Ayerst

Source: Action for Corporate Accountability, 910 17th Street N.W., #413, Washington, D.C., 20006. Phone 202-776-0595; Fax: 202-776-0599.

BOYCOTT NOTE

Nestlé and American Home Products produce a number of infant formulas, including Carnation Good Start, SMA, and Nursoy. These products are not included in the boycott list. Organizers decided that boycotting infant formula would place an unnecessary burden on those who are already victimized by this issue—the mothers.

WAYS TO PARTICIPATE IN THE BOYCOTT

1. Don't buy Nestlé and AHP products.
2. Write to the Nestlé and AHP CEO's and tell them you are boycotting them.
3. Tell your store managers why you are boycotting certain products.
4. Write your members of Congress.
5. Gather signatures on boycott petitions.
6. Form a local boycott group.
7. Set up booths with boycott information at conferences and fairs.
8. Put notices about the boycott in newsletters of organizations that you belong to.
9. Get your organization, church, or business to endorse the boycott.
10. Stop your local school or children's sports organization from using Katherine Beich or Harry Lunden candies for fundraising.
11. Show the video *Formula for Disaster* to friends, in meetings, or on your local Public Access TV channel.
12. Write letters to the editor.
13. Contact Action for product lists, petitions, and other handouts.
14. Send copies of letters and summaries of activities to Action.

Appendix E

U.S. Infant Formulas: Product Ownership

Parent Company	Formula Subsidiary	Formula Brand Names
Abbott Laboratories	Ross Laboratories	Similac, Isomil
American Home Products	Wyeth-Ayerst Laboratories	SMA, S-26, Nursoy
Bristol Myers	Mead Johnson	Enfamil, ProSobee, Gerber
Nestlé	Carnation	Good Start

Appendix F

Physician's Pledge to Protect, Promote, and Support Breastfeeding

RECOGNIZING that breastfeeding plays a uniquely important role in the healthy development of infants and young children;

... that no substitute can provide the complex balance of nutrients, antibodies and growth factors that make breastmilk the perfect food for infants;

... that women have the right to make infant-feeding decisions based on complete and accurate information;

... that my role as a physician is one of influence and responsibility and trust;

... that breastfeeding is an endangered natural resource that requires my protection, promotion and support;

... that current marketing practices -- including the free and low-cost distribution of breastmilk substitute supplies to hospitals and other parts of the health care system -- compete against and discourage breastfeeding;

... that my government, at the 1994 World Health Assembly, affirmed that the marketing and promotion of breastmilk substitutes should not be conducted anywhere in the health care system; and

... that the promotion of health and the prevention of disease are my duties and the mandates of responsible health care providers everywhere;

I, _____ ,

hereby pledge to do my part to protect, promote and support breastfeeding and to work to end the free and low-cost distribution of breastmilk substitutes in our health care systems.

Kindly return to:

Mr. James P. Grant
Physician's Pledge
3 United Nations Plaza
New York, New York 10017
By fax: (212) 303-7911

Please print your full name and address clearly.

_____
_____
_____
_____

Appendix G

Summary of Enacted Breastfeeding Legislation as of March, 1996

Breastfeeding legislation has been enacted in eleven states: Florida, Illinois, Iowa, Michigan, Nevada, New York, North Carolina, Texas, Utah, Wisconsin, and Virginia over the past two years, and many more states have pending bills. The legislation typically clarifies the fact that breastfeeding is not indecent exposure, and thus not criminal behavior. Most of the states have gone further than this, and have made it perfectly clear that a woman has a right to beastfeed anyplace she has a right to be. New York has gone the furthest. New York's law protects the right to breastfeed in public as a mother's civil right!

The legislation is being enacted not because it is currently illegal to beastfeed in public but because it is in the public perception that breastfeeding is indecent exposure. It is hoped that enacting legislation guaranteeing the right to breastfeed in public will help remove just one more stumbling block from a mother's decision to breastfeed. Legislation that recognizes the importance of breastfeeding is just one step toward helping our society become more supportive of breastfeeding.

FL   Senate Bill #472, 1993   Amends many criminal statutes to exclude a mother's breastfeeding her baby; creates a new law stating breastfeeding must be encouraged, and gives a mother a right to breastfeed her baby any place she has the right to be, public or private, even if the nipple is exposed during or incidental to breastfeeding.

FL   Senate Bill #1668, 1994   Creating worksite breastfeeding support policies for all state employees including a demonstration project in Miami to implement the policies; provides for encouragement of breastfeeding in nutrition programs.

IL   Senate Bill #190, 1995   Amends the criminal statutes by stating that breastfeeding of infants is not an act of public indecency.

IA   House File 2350, 1994   Exempts breastfeeding mothers from jury duty who are responsible for the daily care of the child and not regularly employed.

MI   Senate Bills 107–109, 1994   Excludes from the public nudity laws a woman breastfeeding a baby whether or not the nipple or areola is exposed during or incidental to the feeding.

NY   Senate Bill 3999-A, 1994   Creates a new law under the civil rights act that
     gives a mother the right to breastfeed her baby any place she has the right to be,
     public or private, even if the nipple is exposed during or incidental to breast-
     feeding.

NV   Senate Bill 317, 1995   Creates a new law (under Ch. 201 of NRS) that
     states a mother may breastfeed her child in a public or private location where
     the mother is otherwise authorized to be, irrespective of whether the nipple of
     the mother's breast is uncovered during or incidental to the breastfeeding. The
     new law also lays out an updated version of Florida's 1993 bill, giving health
     benefits to mother and baby, recommendations of the AAP, UNICEF and WHO.
     Also amends criminal statutes stating that breastfeeeding of a child by the child's
     mother does not constitue an act of open or gross lewdness, or an act of open
     and indecent or obscene exposure of her body.

NC   Gen. Stat. sec. 14-190.9, 1993   In the indecent exposure statutes, it states
     a woman has a right to breastfeed in any public or private location in which she
     has the right to be, even if the nipple is exposed during or incidental to breast-
     feeding.

TX   House Bill 359, 1995   Creates a new law (Subtitle H, Title 2, Health and
     Safety Code, Chapter 165) stating that breastfeeding a baby is an important and
     basic act and must be encouraged in the interests of maternal and child health
     and family values. The legislature recognizes breastfeeding as the best method of
     infant nutrition, and states a mother is entitled to breastfeed her baby in any
     location in which the mother is authorized to be. This bill also creates a new
     section encouraging breastfeeding in the workplace by allowing businesses that
     develop a policy supporting work-site breastfeeding to use the designation
     "mother-friendly" in promotional materials. Provides that state agencies that ad-
     minister programs providing maternal and child health services shall provide
     information that encourages breastfeeding. Similar to Florida's 1994 bill, it also
     creates worksite breastfeeding support policies for all state employees, including
     a demonstration project to implement policies.

UT   House Bill 262, 1995   Provides that a woman's breastfeeding, including
     breastfeeding in any place where the woman otherwise may rightfully be, does
     not under any circumstances constitute an obscene, lewd, or indecent act, irre-
     spective of whether or not the breast is covered during or incidental to feeding.
     Prevents boards of commissioners, city councils of cities, and county legislative
     bodies from prohibiting a woman's breastfeeding.

VA   Code sec. 18.2-387, 1994   Exempts breastfeeding a child in any public
     place or place where others are present from indecent exposure statute.

VA   House Joint Resolution #248, 1994   Requests the Department of Medical
     Assistance Services to look at including lactation education and supplies for Med-
     icaid recipients. Sets forth benefits of breastfeeding.

Source: Elizabeth Baldwin, J.D., and Kenneth Friedman, J.D., Miami, FL.

References

INTRODUCTION

Baby Milk Action. *Baby Milk Action Update*. Cambridge, England, Issue 10, March 1993.

Baumslag, N. *Breastfeeding: The Passport to Life*. NGO Committee on UNICEF (Working Group on Nutrition), 1989.

Burton, T. "Methods of Marketing Infant Formula Land Abbott in Hot Water." *Wall Street Journal*, May 25, 1993.

Cunningham, A.S., D.B. Jelliffe, and E.F.P. Jelliffe. "Breastfeeding and Health in the 1980s: A Global Epidemiologic Review." *Journal of Pediatrics* 18, (5), May 1991.

FDA Enforcement Report. FDA Press Office, Rockville, MD, June 1994.

Gerlin, A. "A Sandoz Drug Generates a Wave of Lawsuits." *Wall Street Journal*, August 16, 1994.

Hardyment, C. *Dream Babies*. Oxford: Oxford University Press, 1984.

Hormon, E. "Breastfeeding Your Older Child." *Mothering*, Winter 1993.

Kresge, Judy. Personal communication on "Estimate of Percent U.S. Infants Receiving Formula from WIC." Food and Nutrition Service, USDA, October 17, 1994.

INFACT Canada Newsletter. Infant Feeding Action Coalition. Toronto, Canada, Fall 1993.

Jackson, Marni. *The Mother Zone*. New York: Henry Holt, 1994.

Jeffery, C. "Milk Duds." *Washington City Paper*, June 17, 1994.

La Leche League International. *Facts about Breastfeeding*, 1991 and 1994. Center for Breastfeeding Information, La Leche League International, Schaumburg, IL.

Lanting, C.I., V. Fidler, M. Huisman, B.C.L. Touwen, and E.R. Boersma. "The Neurological Differences between 9-year-old Children Fed Breast-Milk or Formula as Babies." *Lancet* 344, 1319, 1994.

Lucas, A., R. Morley, T.J. Cole, G. Lister, and C. Leeson-Payne. "Breast Milk and

Subsequent Intelligence Quotient in Children Born Preterm. *Lancet* 339: 261, 1992.

Nylander, G., R. Lindemann, E. Helsing, and E. Bendvold. "Unsupplemented breastfeeding in the Maternity Ward: Positive Long-Term Effects. *Acta obstertrica Scandinavica* 70, 2055, 1991.

Palmer, G. *The Politics of Breastfeeding.* London: Pandora Press, 1993.

Radford, A. *The Ecological Impact of Bottle Feeding.* Cambridge, England: Baby Milk Action Coalition, 1991.

Victora, C.G. "Evidence for the Protection of Breastfeeding against Infant Deaths from Infectious Diseases in Brazil. *Lancet* 8, August, 1987.

Walker, M. "A Fresh Look at the Risks of Artificial Infant Feeding." *Journal of Human Lactation* 9 (2), 1993.

CHAPTER 1

Aeginata, P. *The Seven Books of Paulus Aeginata*, London: Sydenham Society, 1844.

Apple, R.D., "How Shall I Feed My Baby? Infant Feeding in the United States, 1870–1940." Ph.D. diss., University of Wisconsin—Madison, 1981.

Baldwin, E.N., and K.A. Friedman. "Breastfeeding Legislation in the United States." *New Beginnings*, 164, November–December, 1994.

Baumslag, N. "Breastfeeding: Cultural Practices and Variations." In *Advances in Maternal and Child Health* vol. 7 (edited by D.B. Jelliffe and E.F.P. Jelliffe). Oxford: Oxford University Press, 1987.

Benedict, R. *Patterns of Cultures.* Boston: Houghton Mifflin, 1959.

Budin, P. *The Nursling: The Feeding and Hygiene of Premature and Full Term Infants.* London: Caxton, 1907.

Cadogan, W. *Essay on the Nursing and Management of Children.* London, 1748.

Center for Disease Control. Morbidity and Mortality Reports, 3, 31. Atlanta: CDC, 1982.

Cone, T.E. *History of American Pediatrics.* Boston: Little, Brown, 1979.

Cook, W.H. *Woman's Hand-Book of Health: A Guide for the Wife, Mother and Nurse.* 5th edition. Cincinnati: W.H. Cook, 1866.

Duke-Elder, S. "The History of Ocular Therapeutics." In *System of Ophthalmology.* St. Louis: Mosby, 1962.

Fildes, V. "Neonatal Feeding Practice and Neonatal Mortality during the Eighteenth Century." *Journal of Biosociology* 12, 1980.

Griffin, K. "Good Earth." In *Health Magazine*, May/June 1991.

Hamosh, M., and A. Goldman. *Human Lactation II.* New York: Plenum, 1986.

Jelliffe, D.B., and E.F.P. Jelliffe. *Human Milk in the Modern World.* Oxford: Oxford University Press, 1978.

Kitzinger, S. *Women As Mothers.* Glasgow: Fontana Books, 1978.

Klaus, M.H., and J.H. Kendall. *Maternal Infant Bonding.* St. Louis: Mosby, 1976.

La Leche League International. *The Breastfeeding Answer Book.* Franklin Park, IL: La Leche League International Press, 1991.

Lanting, C.I., V. Fidler, M. Huisman, B.C.L. Touwen, and E.R. Boersma. "The

Neurological Differences between 9-Year-Old Children Fed Breast-Milk or Formula as Babies." *Lancet* 344, 1319, 1994.

Lawrence, R. *Breastfeeding. A Guide for the Medical Profession.* St. Louis: Mosby, 1994.

Lucas, A., R. Morley, T.J. Cole, G. Lister, and C. Leeson-Payne. Breast Milk and Subsequent Intelligence Quotient in Children Born Preterm. *Lancet* 339, 261, 1992

Moser, P.B., R.D. Reynolds, S. Acharya, M.P. Howard, and B. Adon. "Calcium and Magnesium Dietary Intakes and Plasmas and Milk Concentrations of Nepalese Lactating Women." *American Journal of Clinical Nutrition* 47 (4), 735, 1988.

Naeye, R.L., W. Blanc, and C. Paul. "Effects of Maternal Nutrition on the Human Fetus." *Pediatrics* 52, 1973.

Nicholas, R. "Toxic Breasts." *Mother Jones Magazine*, January/February 1992.

Novello, A. "You Can Eat Healthy and Enjoy It." *Parade,* November 11, 1990.

Palmer, G. *The Politics of Breastfeeding.* London: Pandora Press, 1988, 1993.

Phayer, T. *The Regiment of Life.* London: Edward Whitchurche, 1546.

Ploss, H.H., M.C.A. Bartels, and P.R.A. Bartels. Das Weib in der Natur—und Volkerkunde. Brieben: Leipzig, 1885.

Prochownik, C. Cited in Delee, J.B. *The Principles and Practice of Obstetrics.* Philadelphia: W.B. Saunders, 1913.

Radbill, S.X. "Pediatrics in the Bible." *Clinical Pediatrics* 199, 1963.

Raphael, D. *The Tender Gift: Breastfeeding.* Englewood Cliffs, NJ: Prentice-Hall, 1973.

Read, M. *Culture, Health and Disease.* London: Tavistock Publications, 1966.

Rosetta, L. "Breastfeeding and Postpartum Amenorrhea in Sere Women in Senegal." *Annals of Human Biology* 16 (4), 1989.

Scott, S. *Food Beliefs Affecting the Nutritional Status of People in Sierra Leone.* Freetown, Sierra Leone: National School of Nursing, 1978.

Soranus, E. *Gynecology.* Translated by O. Tempkin, N.J. Eastman, L. Edelstein, and A.S. Guttmacher. Baltimore: Johns Hopkins University Press, 1956.

Speert, H. *Iconographia Gyniatria. A Pictorial History of Gynecology and Obstetrics.* Philadelphia: F.A. Davies Company, 1945.

Stanway, P., and A. Stanway. *Breast is Best.* London: Pan Books, 1978.

Steinbeck, J. *Grapes of Wrath.* New York: Viking Penguin Press, 1977.

Thevenin, T. *The Family Bed.* Wayne, NJ: Avery Publishing Group, 1987.

Tomasak, R.L. "A Brief History of the Use of Mother's Milk in Occular Therapeutics." *The Bulletin of the Cleveland Medical Library* 24 (1), 12, 1978.

Vermury, M., and H. Levine. *Project on Beliefs and Practices That Affect Food Habits, A Literature Review.* New York: CARE, 1978.

WHO/UNICEF. *Innocenti Declaration on the Protection, Promotion and Support of Breastfeeding.* Adopted Florence, Italy, August 1, 1990.

Wickes, I.G. *The History of Infant Feeding. Archives of Diseases in Children* 28, 332, 1953.

Yurdakok, K., T. Yazuz, and C.E. Taylor. "Swaddling and Acute Respiratory Infections." *American Journal of Public Health* 80, 7, 1990.

Zhi-chien, H. "Breastfeeding in Xinhui District in South China." *Food and Nutrition Bulletin* 3, 42, 1978.

CHAPTER 2

"Banking on Infant Nourishment." *Mothering*, Summer, 1993.

Blanton, B.W. *Medicine in Virginia in the Eighteenth Century*. Richmond: Garrett and Massie, 1931.

Deaver, J.B., J. McFarland, and J.L. Herman. *The Breast: Its Anomalies, Its Diseases, and Its Treatment*. Philadelphia: Blakstone Son & Co., 1917.

Digby, I., and B. Mathias, *The Joy of the Baby*. Cited in G. Palmer, *The Politics of Breastfeeding*. London: Pandora Press, 1988.

Guerra, F. *American Medical Bibliography, 1639–1783*. New York: Lathrop C. Harper, 1962. As printed in Thomas E. Cone, *History of American Pediatrics*, Boston: Little, Brown, 1979.

Guillemeau, J. (Facsimile edition 1612). *Childbirth or, The Happy Deliverie of Children*. Amsterdam: Theatrum Orbis Terrararum, 1972.

Jelliffe, D.B., and E.F.P. Jelliffe. *Human Milk in the Modern World*. Oxford: Oxford University Press, 1978.

McGee, H. *On Food and Cooking: The Science and Lore of the Kitchen*. New York: Collier Books, 1984.

Mead, M. 1957. Cited in D.B. Jelliffe and E.F.P. Jelliffe. *Human Milk in the Modern World*. Oxford: Oxford University Press, 1978.

Merhav, H.J., Wright, H., Mieles, L.A., and Van Thiel, D.H. "Treatment of IgA Deficiency in Liver Transplant Recipients with Human Breastmilk." *Transplant International* 8, 327, 1995.

Minchin, M. *The Genuine Liebraumilch: A National Treasure at Risk!* Armadale, Australia: Alma Publications, November 1990.

Moffet, T. *Health Improvement*. London: Thomas Newcomb for Samuel Thomson, 1655.

Platt, B.S., and S.Y. Gin. "Chinese Methods of Infantfeeding and Nursing." *Archives of Disease in Children* 13, 343, 1938.

Pliny the Elder. *Natural History*. Oxford: Clarendon Press, 1964.

Ploss, H.H. *Women*. 3 vols. Philadelphia: Heinemann, 1935.

Radbill, S.X. "The Role of Animals in Infant Feeding." In *UCLA Conference on American Folk Medicine (1973): American Folk Medicine, A Symposium*. Edited, with an introduction by W.D. Hand. Los Angeles: University of California Press, 1976.

Schwab, M.G. "The Rise and Fall of the Baby's Bottle." *Journal of Human Nutrition* 33, 276, 1979.

Short, R. "Breastfeeding, Fertility and Population Growth." ACC/SCN Symposium Report, Nutrition Policy Discussion Paper No. 11. ACC/SCN 18th Session Symposium, UNICEF, New York, August 1993.

Sussman, G.D. *Selling Mothers' Milk: The Wet-nursing Business in France, 1715–1914*. Chicago: University of Illinois Press, 1982.

Wickes, I.G. "A History of Infant Feeding." *Archives of Diseases in Children* 28, 1953.

Witkowski, G.J. *Histoire des Accouchements chez Tous les Peuples*. Paris: Steinheil, 1887.

CHAPTER 3

Almroth, S., and P.D. Bidigen "No Need for Water Supplementation for Exclusively Breastfed Infants under Hot, Arid Conditions." *Trans. Roy. Soc. trop. Med. Hyg.* 84, 602, 1990.

Anceschi, M.M., A. Petrelli, G. Zaccardo, A. Barbati, G.C. Renzo, E.V. Cosmi, and M. Hallman. "Inositol and Glucocorticoid in the Development of Lung Stability in Male and Female Rabbit Fetuses." *Pediatric Resident* 24, 1988.

Apple, R.D. "How Shall I Feed My Baby? Infant Feeding in the United States, 1870–1940." Ph.D. diss., University of Wisconsin—Madison, 1981.

Aristotle, *The Complete Works of Aristotle.* Vôl. 1. Princeton, NJ: Princeton University Press, 1978. Cited in R. Short, "Breastfeeding, Fertility and Population Growth." ACC/SCN Symposium Report, Nutrition Policy Discussion Paper No. 11. ACC/SCN 18th Session Symposium, UNICEF, New York, August 1993.

Baby Milk Action. *Baby Milk Action Update.* Cambridge, England, Issue 8, July 1992.

———. Cambridge, England, Issue 11, July 1993.

Baumslag, N. "Do Infants under Six Months of Age Need Extra Iron? A Probe." Working paper no. 12, Mother Care, Arlington, VA, 1992.

Baumslag, N., and P. Putney. *Infant Feeding Patterns, Practices and Trends. Selected Asia/Near East Countries.* Washington, DC: USAID Near East Bureau, May 1989.

Belson, N. Study reported in the *Lancet*, February 1, 1992. Cited in "Children's Higher IQ is Linked to Breast Milk." *Washington Post*, January 31, 1992.

Bronson, G. "Breastfeeding Advocates Increasingly Question Safety, Nutritional Value of Infants' Formulas." *Wall Street Journal*, March 20, 1980.

Brown, D. "Dairies Get an 'F' for Vitamin D Content." *Washington Post*, April 30, 1992.

Bruce, R.C., and H.M. Kliegman. "Hyponatremic Seizures among Infants Fed with Commercial Bottled Drinking Water." *Morbidity and Mortality Weekly Report* 43, 35, September 9, 1994.

Clavano, N. "The Results of Change in Hospital Practices. A Pediatrician's Campaign for Breastfeeding in the Philippines." *Assignment Children* 55/56, 1981.

Cotton, A.C. *Care of Children.* Chicago: American School of Home Economics, 1907.

Cunningham, A.S., D.B. Jelliffe, and E.F.P. Jelliffe. *Breastfeeding, Growth and Illness: An Annotated Bibliography.* New York: UNICEF, 1992.

———. "Breast-Feeding and Health in the 1980s: A Global Epidemiological Review." *The Journal of Pediatrics* 68, 1991.

Ebrahim, G.J. "The Contraceptive Effect of Breastfeeding—An Update." *Journal of Tropical Pediatrics* 37, 210, 1991.

Gerlin, A. "A Sandoz Drug Generates a Wave of Lawsuits." *Wall Street Journal*, August 16, 1994.

Hallman, M., K. Bry, K. Hoppu, M. Lappi, and M. Pojavuori. "Inositol Supplementation in Premature Infants with Respiratory Distress Syndrome." *New England Journal of Medicine* 326, 1992.

Hambraeus, L. "Proprietary Milks versus Human Breast Milk. A Critical Approach from the Nutritional Point of View." *Pediatric Clinics of North America* 24, 17, 1977.

Howie, W., J.S. Forsyth, S.A. Ogston, A. Clark, and C.D. Florey. "Protective Effect of Breastfeeding against Infection." *British Medical Journal* 300, 6716, 11, January 6, 1990.

Humane Society. "BGH Causes National Brouhaha." *Humane Society of the United States News*, Spring 1994.

Institute of Medicine. *Nutrition during Lactation*. Washington, DC: National Academy Press, 1991.

Jansson, E. *Petition for a Breast Milk Purity Strategy*. Washington, DC: National Network to Prevent Birth Defects, March 1985.

Jeffery, C. "Milk Duds." *Washington City Paper*, June 17, 1994.

Kennedy, K.I., R. Rivera, and A.S. McNeilly. "Consensus Statement on the Use of Breastfeeding as a Family Planning Method. *Contraception*, 39 (5), 1989.

King, F.S. *Helping Mothers Breastfeed*. Rev. ed. Nairobi, Kenya: AMREF, 1993.

Knodel, J., and E. van der Walle. "Breast Feeding, Fertility and Infant Mortality." *Population Studies* 21, 1967.

Labbok, M.M. "Breastfeeding and Contraception." Letter in *New England Journal of Medicine*, 308 (1), 51, 1983.

Lawrence, R.A. *Breastfeeding: A Guide for the Medical Profession*. Princeton, NJ: Mosby, 1994.

Lonnerdal, B. "Effects of Oral Contraceptive Agents upon Lactation." International Workshop on Human Lactation, Maternal-Environmental Factors, Oahaca, Mexico, January 15–19, 1986.

Mason, M. "Milk? It May Not Do a Body Good." *Washington Post*, March 7, 1994.

Mayer, C. "Milk Takes a Spill." *The Washington Post*, February 6, 1991.

Minchin, M. *The Genuine Liebfraumilch: A National Treasure at Risk!* Armadale, Australia: Alma Publications, November 1990.

Mohrbacher, N., and J. Stock. *The Breastfeeding Answer Book*. Franklin Park, IL: La Leche League International, 1991.

Palmer, G. *The Politics of Breastfeeding*. London: Pandora Press, 1994.

Pereira, G.R., L. Baker, J. Egler, L. Corcoran, and R. Chiavacci. "Serum Myoinsitol Concentrations in Premature Infants Fed Human Milk, Formula for Infants, and Parenteral Nutrition." *American Journal of Clinical Nutrition* 51, 1990.

Radford, A. *The Ecological Impact of Bottle Feeding*. London: Baby Milk Action, 1991.

Riordan, J., and K. Auerbach. *Breastfeeding and Human Lactation*. Boston: Jones and Barlett.

Rogan, W.J., A. Bagniewska, and T. Damstra. "Pollutants in Breast Milk." *New England Journal of Medicine*, 302 (26), 1980.

Rosen, G. *A History of Public Health*. New York: MD Publications, 1958.

Rotch, T.M. *The Hygienic and Medical Treatment of Children*. Philadelphia: Lippincott, 1895.

Ruff, A.J. "Breast Milk, Breastfeeding and Transmission of Viruses to the Neonate." *Seminars in Perinatology* 18 (6), 510, 1994.

Salisbury, I., and A.G. Blackwell. *Petition to Alleviate Domestic Infant Formula Misuse and Provide Informed Infant Feeding Choice.* San Francisco: Public Advocates Inc., 1982. As cited in M.A. Walker. "A Fresh Look at the Risks of Artificial Infant Feeding." *Journal of Human Lactation* 9 (2), 1993.

Semba, R.D., P.G. Miotti, J.D. Chipangwi, A.J. Saah, J.K. Canner, G.A. Dallabeth, and D.R. Hoover. "Maternal Vitamin A Deficiency and Mother-to-Child Transmission of HIV-1." *Lancet* 343, 1593, 1994.

Sepkoski, C.M., B.M. Lester, G.W. Ostheimer, and T.B. Brazelton. "The Effects of Maternal Epidural Anesthesia on Neonatal Behavior during the First Month." *Developmental Medicine and Child Neurology* 34, 1072, 1992.

Short, R. "Breastfeeding, Fertility and Population Growth," ACC/SCN Symposium Report, Nutrition Policy Discussion Paper No. 11. ACC/SCN 18th Session Symposium, UNICEF, New York, August 1993.

Vis, H.D., and P.H. Hennart. "The Decline in Breastfeeding." *Acta Pediatrica Belg.* 31, 195, 1978.

Walker, M. "A Fresh Look at the Risks of Artificial Infant Feeding." *Journal of Human Lactation* 9 (2), 1993.

Wolfe, S., M. Jones, and R. Donkin. *Women's Health Alert.* New York: Addison-Wesley, 1991.

CHAPTER 4

Apple, R.D. "How Shall I Feed My Baby? Infant Feeding in the United States, 1870–1940." Ph.D. diss., University of Wisconsin—Madison, 1981.

Auerbach, K. "One Result of Marketing: Breastfeeding Is the Exception in Infant Feeding." Editorial. *Journal of Tropical Pediatrics* 38 (5), 210–213, 1992.

Baumslag, N. "Breastfeeding: The Passport to Life." NGO Committee on UNICEF, New York, 1989.

Berg, A. *The Nutrition Factor.* Washington, DC: The Brookings Institution, 1973.

Cone, T.E. *The History of American Pediatrics.* Boston: Little, Brown, 1978.

Cotton, A.C. *Care of Children.* Chicago: American School of Home Economics, 1907.

Drake, T.G. "Infant Feeders and Feeding in Bygone Days." *Chemist and Druggist Annual Special Issue,* 1956.

Ebrahim, G.J. *Breast Feeding: The Biological Option.* London: Macmillan, 1979.

Fildes, V.A. *Breasts, Bottles and Babies: A History of Infant Feeding.* Edinburgh: Edinburgh University Press, 1986.

Jelliffe, D. As cited in Walker, M. "A Fresh Look at the Risks of Artificial Infant Feeding." *Journal of Human Lactation* 9 (2), 1993.

Knodel, J., and E. van der Walle. "Breast Feeding, Fertility and Infant Mortality." *Population Studies* 21, 109, September 1967.

Lawrence, R.A. *Breastfeeding: A Guide for the Medical Profession.* St. Louis, MO: Mosby, 1994.

Palmer, G. From "Breastmilk: A world resource." Presented at La Leche League International's 35th Conference, Miami Beach, Florida, July 24–27, 1991.

————. *The Politics of Breastfeeding*. London: Pandora Press, 1994.

Radford, A. *The Ecological Impact of Bottle Feeding*. Cambridge, England: Baby Milk Action Coalition, 1991.

Rosen, G. *A History of Public Health*. New York: MD Publications, 1958.

Schwab, M.G. "The Rise and Fall of the Baby's Bottle." *Journal of Human Nutrition* 33, 276, 1979.

Short, R. "Breastfeeding, Fertility and Population Growth." ACC/SCN Symposium Report, Nutrition Policy Discussion Paper No. 11. ACC/SCN 18th Session Symposium, UNICEF, New York, August 1993.

Spock, B. "In the Doctor's Opinion." *Parenting*, September 1992.

Strauss, L. *Diseases in Milk*. 2d ed. New York: Dutton, 1917.

Wickes, I.G. "A History of Infant Feeding." *Archives of Diseases in Children* 28, 1953.

Zimbabwe Ministry of Health. "Baby Feeding and Towards a Health Model for Zimbabwe." Harare, Zimbabwe: Ministry of Health. Funded by UNICEF, 1981.

CHAPTER 5

Baby Milk Action. *Government Interference, Baby Milk Action Update*. Cambridge, England: October 12, 1993.

————. *So little for So Much, Baby Milk Action Update*. Cambridge, England, October 12, 1993.

Burton, T. "Methods of Marketing Infant Formula Land Abbott in Hot Water." *Wall Street Journal*, May 25, 1993.

Consumer Reports. "The Sour Tale of Baby Formula Pricing." *Consumer Reports*, October 1993.

Day, K. "In Health Care, Pay Outpaces Perception." *Washington Post*, March 31, 1993.

Jeffery, C. "Milk Duds." *Washington City Paper*, June 17, 1994.

Kresge, J. Personal communication on "Estimate of Percent U.S. Infants Receiving Formula from WIC." Food and Nutrition Service, USDA, October 17, 1994.

Margolis, L.H. "The Ethics of Accepting Gifts from Pharmaceutical Companies." *Pediatrics* 88 (6), 1991. As cited in *Breastfeeding Briefs*, 16, IBFAN, Penang, Malaysia, September 1992.

Palmer, G. *The Politics of Breastfeeding*. London: Pandora Press, 1994.

Radford, A., and M. Arts. *Breaking the Rules: 1991*. Cambridge: International Baby Food Action Network, 1991.

Sturmer, K. *Action News*. Action for Corporate Accountability, Fall 1993 and Summer 1994.

"Switch, Clinton Supports Infant Formula Code." *Daily Citizen* 1 (70), May 10, 1994.

Tanouye, E. "Drug Companies' Marketing Practices Affect Doctors' Behavior, Study Finds." *Wall Street Journal*, March 2, 1994.

Testimony before the Subcommittee on Antitrust, Monopolies, and Business Rights, Senate Judiciary Committee, May 29, 1990.

Testimony before the Texas Department of Health, December 30, 1987.

Walker, M. "A Fresh Look at the Risks of Artificial Infant Feeding." *Journal of Human Lactation* 9 (2), 1993.

Wall Street Journal, "Nestlé Unit Sues Baby Formula Firms, Alleging Conspiracy with Pediatricians." *Wall Street Journal,* June 1, 1993.

WHO/UNICEF. *Innocenti Declaration on the Protection, Promotion and Support of Breastfeeding.* Adopted Florence Italy, August 1, 1990.

WHO/UNICEF. *The WHO/UNICEF International Code of Marketing Breastmilk Substitutes.* WHA Geneva, Switzerland, May 1981.

Williams, C.D. "Milk and Murder." Address to the Singapore Rotary Club, 1939, edited by A. Allain (1986), International Organization of Consumers' Unions, P.O. Box 1045, 10830 Penang, Malaysia.

Williams, C.D., N.B. Baumslag, and D.B. Jelliffe. *Mother and Child Health: Delivering the Services.* New York: Oxford University Press, 1994.

CHAPTER 6

Clearinghouse on Infant Feeding and Maternal Nutrition. "Government Legislation and Policies to Support Breastfeeding, Improve Maternal and Infant Nutrition, and Implement a Code of Marketing of Breastmilk Substitutes. Report No. 5. Washington DC: American Public Health Association, 1988.

Farber, E., M. Alejandro-Wright, and S. Muenchow. "Infant Care Leave Survey." Yale Bush Center in Child Development and Social Policy, Infant Care Leave Project, Summaries of Research Components, 1983–1985, Yale University, 1986.

Lopata, P. "Government Policies and Babies." *Mothering,* Winter 1993.

"Odds and Ends." *Wall Street Journal,* April 8, 1994.

Smolowe, J. "Where Children Come First," *Time,* November 9, 1992.

Star, M.G. "Flexibility in Corporate America." *Mothering,* Summer 1993.

Tousignant, M. "When Nursing Moms Go Back to Work." *Washington Post,* November 6, 1993.

Von Esterik, P. "Women, Work and Breastfeeding." Cornell International Nutrition, Series No. 23, Cornell University, Ithaca, New York, 1992.

Waring, M. *If Women Counted: A New Feminist Economics.* New York: Harper and Row, 1988.

Williams, C. "Milk and Murder." Address to the Singapore Rotary Club, 1939, edited by A. Allain (1986), International Organization of Consumers' Unions, P.O. Box 1045, 10830 Penang, Malaysia.

Wolf, N. *The Beauty Myth.* New York: Anchor Books, 1992.

Women's Bureau. "Facts on Working Women." U.S. Department of Labor, No. 93–2, June 1993.

Index

About the Authors

NAOMI BAUMSLAG, M.D., M.P.H., is Clinical Professor of Pediatrics at Georgetown University Medical School in Washington, DC, and president of the Women's International Public Health Network in Bethesda, MD. She has served as an advisor to USAID, UNICEF, WHO, the Georgia Department of Human Resources, PAHO, and the governments of many developing countries as well as the Health Council of the La Leche League International (LLLI) and the World Alliance of Breastfeeding Associations (WABA). The author of more than 100 articles and eight books, Dr. Baumslag lectures widely both nationally and internationally.

DIA L. MICHELS is a science writer whose articles and essays have appeared in newspapers and magazines around the world. Her commitment to breastfeeding has come both from her research and from her experience nursing her own children over the past six years. This is the second book she has written with Dr. Baumslag. *A Woman's Guide to Yeast Infections* was published in 1992.